Your Offshore Doctor

Your Offshore Doctor

A Manual of
Medical Self-Sufficiency at Sea

Dr. Michael H. Beilan

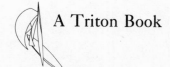

A Triton Book

Dodd, Mead & Company • New York

Library of Congress Cataloging-in-Publication Data

Beilan, Michael H.
  Your offshore doctor.

  Bibliography: p.
  Includes index.
    1. Boats and boating—Accidents and injuries—Handbooks, manuals, etc.   2.
First aid in illness and injury—Handbooks, manuals, etc.   3. Medical emergen-
cies—Handbooks, manuals, etc.   4. Medicine, Naval —Handbooks, manuals,
etc. I. Title. [DNLM: 1. Emergencies—handbooks. 2. First Aid—hand-
books.   3. Naval Medicine—handbooks.   WB 39   B422y]
RC88.9B6B45   1985   616'.025   85-13156
ISBN 0-396-08680-2 (pbk.)

This book is dedicated with love to my daughter, Jennifer Sara, whose eyes and smile are a landfall to this seaman.

Contents

Contents

Contents

Contents

Contents

Contents

Introduction

Several years ago, I provisioned my sailboat, *Starship*, for an extended offshore voyage from Hermosa Beach, California, to my prospective new cruising home in the state of Washington. Since I am a physician specializing in emergency care, I especially wanted a well-provisioned medical kit, able to provide not only for the needs of my immediate crew, but any others who might require assistance. When it came to buying a book about medical care at sea, I found that while there were a number of references available on first aid, no text adequately explained what to do when medical care is simply unavailable, or, at best, delayed by several days. This text addresses that problem.

Fortunately, most medical problems are not life-threatening. However, some simple conditions do progress in severity and become dangerous if they are not treated promptly and effectively. In this text, I have not tried to make medical professionals out of those of you who aren't. I have, however, tried to point out what has to get done in a specific medical situation when a crew member ends up functioning as the ship's physician. My aim is to lighten that responsibility by presenting information in simple language, not the complicated medical jargon most people don't understand. Since you can't treat someone without knowing what it is you're dealing with, a step-by-step explanation on how to arrive at a diagnosis is also given.

Many conditions are obvious, or you may have a pretty good idea what it is you're dealing with. In that case, refer to the index to find references to a specific condition. Some problems, such as abdominal pain, various infections, trauma of various kinds, etc., will require you to narrow down your diagnosis in order to arrive at the best treatment. I have attempted to explain clearly the areas I feel it will be important for you to know when you're at sea, whether you're a commercial fisherman or seaman, or a pleasure boater.

Much of the information presented here, dealing with treatment and procedures, is not benign. The medicines used can be dangerous, as can some of the procedures indicated. In a life-and-death situation, there is often no way to avoid these complexities. Appropriate precautions are explained whenever necessary to prevent complications and side effects; however, these sometimes occur. No guarantee of desired results is implied in this text.

The medical kit I've outlined is a comprehensive one. I realize that many people do not have the room aboard, or may not want to spend the money necessary to purchase these items. Obviously, the medical kit aboard a boat making a transoceanic passage will be different from one aboard a weekend cruiser. In either case, though, the kit should meet the boat's needs. Some of you may feel that by not having the appropriate equipment or medicines aboard, you have abrogated your responsibilities to care for someone. I can only say that incomplete preparation will not make any problem go away—you'll still have to deal with someone's suffering in an emergency situation, and indeed their life may depend on your knowledge and acquired skills.

The conditions of wind and sea that most often produce accidents and injuries—steep, confused waves and heavy winds—are also the most difficult conditions in which to provide medical treatment. At times, the acting physician on board may be forced to delay treatment in order to avoid further injury to the patient. An obvious example would be a decision to keep pressure bandages applied to a severe laceration until conditions are calm enough to suture the wound neatly and effectively. It might also be wisest to delay the resetting of a fractured bone until the acting physician is reasonably sure that his treatment in rough weather will not cause extra trauma to the patient. These decisions are difficult, and can only be reached after a consideration of all the factors involved in an emergency situation.

Above all, stay calm and use common sense. Often, professional medical assistance is available by radio or by direct ship-to-ship contact with medical personnel.

I've included a dental section which, although not directly related to the core material in this text, provides simple measures for taking care of dental disorders when no dentist is available.

I hope you will never need to refer to this manual because of an actual medical emergency on board; but if you do, I think you will find its information valuable. The more familiar you are with the information *before* an emergency occurs, the better prepared you will be to minimize its consequences.

Good sailing,
Michael H. Beilan

Acknowledgments

Thanks go to my many friends and crew members who prodded me to answer their health-related questions patiently and in easily understood terms.

In addition to Susan Gilbert, who supplied graphic artwork, illustrations, and psychic energy, the following people graciously gave of their time and made helpful suggestions during the writing of this book:

—Tom Wood, Karen Wood, Trish Gerard: manuscript review

—Leah Owens: typing and manuscript review

—Steve Scharf, D.D.S.: preparation of the dental section

—Susan Beilan, my Ketiah Lady: patience, love, and understanding

Your Offshore Doctor

1. Preparation

1.1 Record Keeping

It is very important that the date, time of injury, condition of the crew member, and response to treatment be accurately recorded and updated (hourly, if possible) in the log. This is not only a medical record, but also a legal one.

The more detailed the record, the better. Any medications given, the time given, how it was given (orally or by injection), and the dosage should all be recorded.

Any preexisting medical conditions should be noted. A general medical exam and physician's checkup should precede all planned offshore voyages of long duration. The pertinent medical background of all crew members should be made available to the captain, and vice versa. Anyone who takes medications for specific illnesses should plan to have good supplies (plus spares) of such medications with them.

1.2 Immunizations

At present, advice from the World Health Organization and the U.S. Center for Disease Control (CDC) indicates that a *tetanus* booster is effective for ten (10) years.*

Appropriate immunization requirements of foreign countries may be obtained from your doctor or the consulate of the country you intend to visit.

Reference text: Foreign Travel Immunization Guide

1

Documentation of all immunizations is necessary and should be kept alongside your passport.

The CDC also publishes a pamphlet called "Health Information for International Travel," which is updated annually and advises on the various diseases endemic in areas worldwide.

1.3 What to Learn Before You Leave

In most communities, the American Heart Association sponsors courses on the principles of basic cardiac life support, invaluable training for any situation demanding cardiopulmonary resuscitation (CPR).

Other organizations, such as the Boy Scouts of America, the American Red Cross, and many community schools and colleges offer first-aid courses that cover the recognition and treatment of minor, non–life-threatening emergencies. Several private organizations, such as Offshore Medical Services (P.O. Box 427, Tarpon Springs, FL 34286-0427), offer information specifically designed for the offshore sailor, covering survival medicine and techniques to enhance medical self-sufficiency at sea.

The object of all this training is to broaden your capabilities and experience, and prepare you to deal with an immediate medical situation, whether minor or severe. I would urge you to explore the resources available in your community and take the time to attend at least one course. This manual should serve to supplement your basic knowledge of various medical conditions, their diagnoses, and their treatments.

1.4 How to Take a Medical History

Although we're usually dealing with an immediate problem, a crew member's past medical history may be important if it has a bearing on that current situation. For example, someone with a food allergy may forget about a previous unpleasant reaction and sit down to a feast of clams, shrimp, or oysters, only to have a repeat allergic reaction, perhaps more severe than the first.

When we ask questions about someone's past history, it's best to categorize these questions and list them, as in the following example:

1. Illnesses, especially any that required hospitalization
2. Operations
3. Allergies to medicines, food, insects, etc.
4. Immunizations
5. Permanent disabilities or disfigurement

In the hospital, I usually review the various organ systems as I question a patient, making notes about any problem the patient has now or has had before. These systems include:

1. Head, eyes, ears, nose, and throat
2. Heart
3. Lungs
4. Stomach and intestines
5. Kidneys and bladder; prostate or menstrual problems
6. Muscles and nerves
7. Skin

Don't be afraid to ask personal questions, but be gentle and compassionate about it.

1.5 How to Perform a Physical Exam

In most cases of minor trauma, a complete physical examination is unnecessary. However, in many situations, such as head trauma, chest pain, abdominal pain, or major trauma, a complete exam is mandatory. An orderly progression from head to toe (similar to taking a medical history, above) will simplify matters and promote thoroughness. Try to pay attention to details, and be sure to record all your findings.

The following list should cover many of the things you're looking for:

1. Appearance: How does the patient look?
2. Vital signs: blood pressure (BP), pulse, respiration, temperature.
3. Eyes: Are the pupils equal? Do they both react when you shine a flashlight in the eyes? Is there any redness or discharge present?
4. Ears: Is there any discharge or bleeding present? Is there a loss of hearing when you whisper to the patient?
5. Nose: Is there any discharge or bleeding present?
6. Throat: Is there any soreness, redness; are there areas of pus in the tonsil area or in the back of the throat? Is there heavy postnasal drip? What is the condition of the gums and teeth? Is there any odor to the breath?
7. Heart: Put your ear over the patient's chest to listen to the heart, or take the patient's pulse. Do the heartbeats feel or sound strong or weak? Is the pulse strong and regular, or weak and thready?
8. Lungs: Can the patient breathe easily? Is there any noise (gurgling or wheezing) when a deep breath is taken?
9. Abdomen: Is there any pain or tenderness? If so, where is it and how severe do you judge it

Preparation

to be? Is there any visible mass, or one that you can feel, in the abdomen or groin region?

10. Genitalia: Is there any pain, redness, or swelling present?
11. Rectal: Are hemorrhoids present? If so, is there bleeding? Are impacted feces present (perhaps because of severe constipation)?
12. Musculoskeletal: Is there any pain or tenderness on movement of fingers or toes, arms or legs? Is any obvious deformity present? Is there back pain or muscle spasms of the neck or back?
13. Skin: Note the skin color, and any obvious abrasion, laceration, or bruise.

Note: The above list is not a complete one, though it provides the basic questions that should be answered.

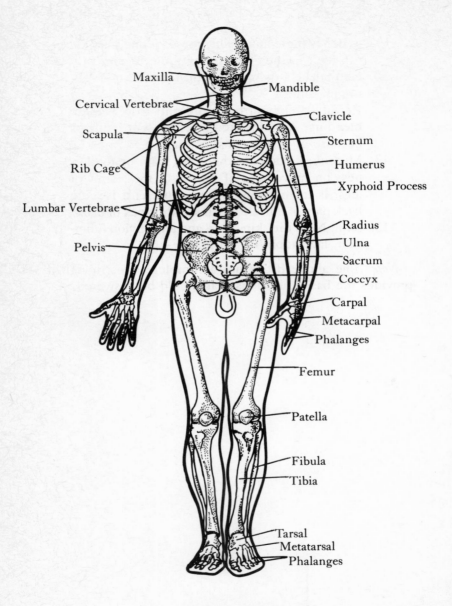

Maxilla

Mandible

Cervical Vertebrae

Clavicle

Scapula

Sternum

Rib Cage

Humerus

Xyphoid Process

Lumbar Vertebrae

Radius

Pelvis

Ulna

Sacrum

Coccyx

Carpal

Metacarpal

Phalanges

Femur

Patella

Fibula

Tibia

Tarsal

Metatarsal

Phalanges

Skeletal system

6

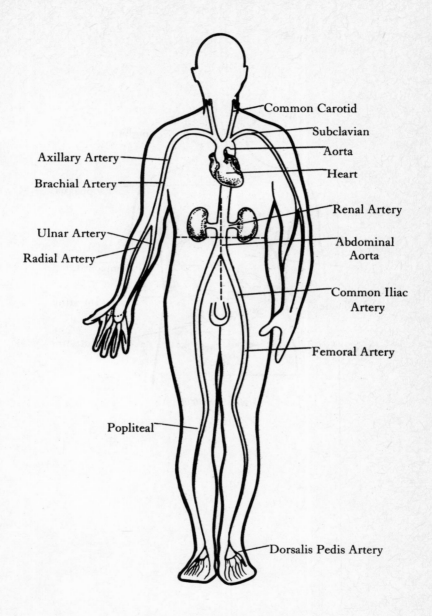

Common Carotid

Subclavian

Aorta

Heart

Axillary Artery

Brachial Artery

Renal Artery

Ulnar Artery

Abdominal
Aorta

Radial Artery

Common Iliac
Artery

Femoral Artery

Popliteal

Dorsalis Pedis Artery

Major arterial circulatory system

7

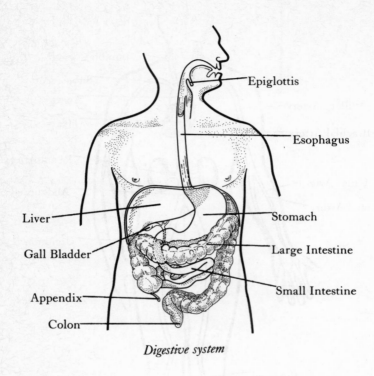

Epiglottis

Esophagus

Liver

Stomach

Gall Bladder

Large Intestine

Small Intestine

Appendix

Colon

Digestive system

2. Lifesaving

2.1 Cardiopulmonary Resuscitation (CPR)

Cardiac arrest may occur as a result of drowning, heart attack, accidents, electric shock, etc.

SIGNS AND SYMPTOMS:
1. The person is not breathing.
2. No pulse can be felt in the neck region or groin.
3. No heartbeat can be heard.
4. The pupils of the eyes may be dilated and non-reactive to light.

The above criteria can be determined in several moments. It is important to keep the blood circulating by resuscitation measures, which must be started within 4–6 minutes after circulation has stopped, or brain damage will occur.

Remember the ABC's of resuscitation:
A = Airway
B = Breathing by artificial ventilation
C = Circulation by artificial means (external cardiac compression)

TO ADMINISTER CPR:
1. Clean the mouth of mucus, blood, or any obstruction.
2. Elevate the chin and pinch off the nose with your thumb and index finger.

9

3. Take a big breath and give the patient two rapid breaths.
4. Locate the lower part of the patient's sternum (breastbone) and keep your fingers and hands above that region. Correct position should be the width of two fingers above the lower tip of the sternum.
5. Place the heel of one hand over the back of the other hand, and, leaning forward so that your shoulders are over the patient's chest, push straight down 1½–2 inches, keeping the elbows straight, for about ½ second, then release. This compresses the heart against the spine, thereby mechanically pushing blood out of the heart and through the body's vessels.
6. The rate of compression and ventilation depends on whether there are one or two rescuers present.

> One person: Compress the chest 15 times, then give two ventilations.
> Two people: Perform from opposite sides of the patient. Give one ventilation after every 5 heart compressions.

7. Continue until the patient resumes breathing independently, or until there has been no reasonable response to resuscitation attempts. Recheck for spontaneous breathing, heartbeat, and carotid (neck) and femoral (groin) pulses.

Note: It is always a difficult decision to stop resuscitation attempts. With the exception of hypothermia victims who drown (see 12.3—"Hypothermia"), patients without oxygenated blood for over six minutes are considered irreversibly brain-damaged. Again, an American Heart Association course in Basic Life Support is offered in most communities, and is invaluable training if a lifesaving situation should arise.

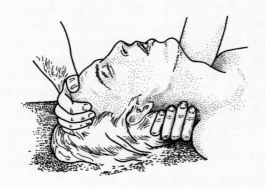

CPR—position of head and neck

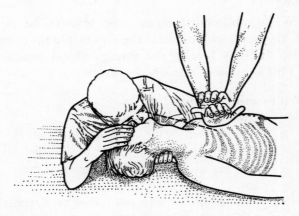

With the head and neck position maintained, the victim is given mouth to mouth resuscitation. Hands should be properly positioned on the sternum. Use the heel of the hand as shown. During ventilation, watch to see that the victim's chest rises when a breath is given.

Your Offshore Doctor

2.2 Choking

The universal distress signal of choking is encircling the throat with one or both hands.

Obstruction of the airway by a foreign object most often occurs during eating. Large pieces of food are often aspirated (breathed in) instead of being properly chewed and swallowed. This is known to occur particularly after alcoholic consumption. Airway obstruction may be either partial or complete, the latter causing death by asphyxiation in several minutes if the obstruction is not removed. You have to react quickly.

SIGNS AND SYMPTOMS:

The victim is unable to talk, cough, or breathe if there is a complete airway obstruction.

TREATMENT:

Perform the abdominal thrust, also referred to as the *Heimlich Maneuver*, which causes the victim's lungs to expel air rapidly, thereby forcing the foreign object out of the airway. This is done in one of two positions:

1. With victim standing:
   a. Stand behind the victim.
   b. Encircle both your arms around the victim's upper abdomen just below the rib cage, *but not on the lower border of the breastplate.*
   c. Holding one fist with your other hand, press the thumb side of your fist rapidly and forcefully upward and into the victim's abdomen. Repeat four times.
   d. If the piece of food is expelled, get ready to remove it from the victim's mouth.

e. If airway obstruction remains unrelieved, CPR may be necessary; see section 2.1.

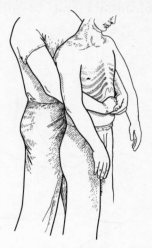

Heimlich maneuver—victim standing. Note position of rescuer's hands.

2. With victim lying on his back:
   a. Position yourself alongside of, or straddling, the victim.
   b. Place the heel of your hand on the victim's upper abdomen, *not on the lower border of the breastplate.* The fingers should point toward the victim's head.
   c. Place your other hand across the top of your first hand.
   d. Keep an upright position, with your shoulders directly over the victim's chest.
   e. Quickly and forcefully thrust downward four times; this should expel the foreign object.
   f. Again, be ready to remove whatever foreign matter comes up into the victim's mouth.

g. If unsuccessful, repeat this maneuver a second or third time.

h. If still unsuccessful, begin CPR (section 2.1).

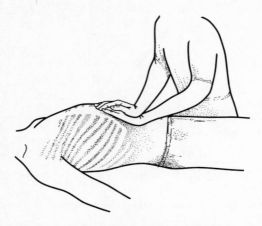

Heimlich maneuver—victim on back. Head is turned to the side. Note position of rescuer's hands below the xyphoid process.

2.3 Bleeding and Shock

Although shock is in itself not a disease, but a result of complex underlying body functions gone awry, I have chosen to include it along with bleeding because hemorrhage is the most common cause of shock. Since our circulating blood volume is necessary for tissue oxygenation and nutrition, when a severe hemorrhage occurs, a corresponding reduction in our blood volume results. Our objectives, then, are to control bleeding and maintain an adequate circulating blood volume before shock sets in.

Stay calm when you see someone bleeding (or in any other emergency situation). At times, the smallest cuts will bleed profusely, making it appear that the victim is hemorrhaging severely; often, this is not the case.

SIGNS AND SYMPTOMS:

Quickly assess the victim. Look for the following, in approximate order of increasing severity:

1. Cool, clammy skin
2. Sweating
3. Dizziness
4. Ashen appearance
5. Rapid pulse
6. Reduced blood pressure
7. Increased thirst
8. Decreased urinary output (a late sign)

Ultimately, if hemorrhage continues unchecked, decreased brain function and death may occur.

TREATMENT:

1. Cut away clothing to permit a complete examination.
2. Perform CPR if necessary.
3. Elevate the feet 12 inches to improve circulation to the heart and brain.
4. Apply direct pressure over the bleeding area.
5. If arterial bleeding is suspected, look for regular spurting of blood from the wound area; this will be synchronous with the heartbeat. Use direct pressure over the area for approximately ten minutes. Apply gauze compresses, 4 × 4-inch bandages, or, as an immediate but less sterile measure, any article of clothing or your bare hand, in a steady pressure over the site.
6. Pressure points and tourniquets should *not* be necessary and are dangerous—limbs have been

15

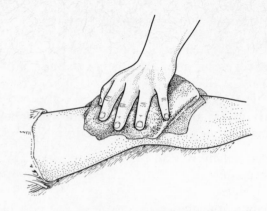

Pressure bandage—use direct pressure over the bleeding site.

lost from overzealous application of tourniquets. Rarely, a tourniquet may have to be used, as when an arm or leg is amputated; but, as a general rule, avoid their use.

7. If bleeding has been severe enough for shock due to hypovolemia (decreased blood volume) to occur, begin an intravenous (IV) infusion with lactated Ringer's solution. Give IV fluids at a rate that will result in clinical improvement. (See sections 15.1 and 15.2 in "Procedures.")

8. Record the victim's blood pressure, pulse, skin color, and urinary output every 15–30 minutes to determine whether clinical improvement is taking place. If urinary output falls to less than 40 cc per hour, and the pulse rate is increasing, more IV fluids are needed at a faster rate.

9. Maintain the victim's body temperature; try to prevent too much accumulation or loss of heat.

2.4 Anaphylactic Shock

Anaphylactic shock is a severe, generalized allergic reaction to one of the following:

16

1. Medications, such as penicillin or horse serum
2. Foods, such as shellfish or berries
3. Insect stings from bees, wasps, etc.
4. Inhaled substances, such as pollens

SIGNS AND SYMPTOMS:

1. Respiratory distress; wheezing, difficulty breathing. This is the most important symptom, as it is the most dangerous to the victim.
2. Hives
3. Itching or burning of the skin, especially of the head and neck region
4. Nausea, vomiting, or diarrhea may occur.
5. Cardiovascular collapse may occur, leading to shock and possibly death.

TREATMENT:

1. Perform CPR if necessary; see section 2.1
2. Administer epinephrine, 1:1000 solution, in a dose of 0.3–0.5 cc subcutaneously. An alternative would be an intramuscular (IM) injection. (See sections 15.3 and 15.4 in "Procedures.") Epinephrine, in the same dose as above, may be repeated every 15–20 minutes for another 1–2 injections.
3. An antihistamine, such as Benadryl, 50 mg IM, may be administered. With recovery, oral Benadryl may be given, in a dose of 25 mg 3–4 times daily for 1–2 days.

PREVENTION:

1. Prevention is not always possible, as someone may react to a food or medication source that

was previously tolerated without ill effect.

2. For known allergies, desensitization injections are advisable.
3. For people known to be sensitive to bee stings, carry a bee-sting kit aboard.

3. Treatment of Infection

3.1 The Meaning of Fever and Its Treatment

Fever is usually a sign of infection, dehydration, or sunstroke. It is only dangerous when it is high. For most patients, this means a temperature of over 103 degrees orally or 104 degrees rectally. It may be dangerous for patients who have had convulsions in the past, because convulsions may reoccur when the temperature gets too high (105 degrees) too fast. The pulse rate usually goes up ten beats per minute for every one degree fahrenheit in elevation of the temperature. The objective of treatment is to try to keep the temperature from getting too high, but if it exceeds safe limits in spite of your efforts, the patient should be sponged off with lukewarm water. See below for further measures.

TREATMENT:

1. Give aspirin regularly. Other fever medicines like Tylenol (acetaminophen) can be used instead. Use proper doses as instructed on the label until the fever is down to 101–102 degrees or less. Tylenol can be alternated with aspirin every two hours (i.e., aspirin at 1400 hours, Tylenol at 1600 hours, aspirin at 1800 hours). Both Tylenol and aspirin have side effects detrimental to various organ systems when given in too high a dosage, so exercise care and keep appropriate records.
2. Encourage consumption of lots of fluids. Drink-

ing fluids is good because there is extra fluid loss from the body during periods of fever. Cool liquids are best. Food is not important; appetite will return later.

3. Use light clothing and covers; this allows body heat to escape. An extra blanket may be added when the patient is chilly, but remove it after the chill has passed. Keep cabin temperature normal if possible.
4. Keep the patient quietly occupied and encourage rest. Too much activity can elevate the temperature.

If the temperature goes over 103–104 degrees rectally in spite of treatment, bathe the patient in lukewarm or cool water until the temperature is reduced to a more reasonable level (101–102 degrees). The water should never be so cold as to cause shivering. If no shower or tub is available, use wet towels to sponge the patient, changing towels as they become warm.

3.2 Eye, Ear, Nose, and Throat Infections

3.2a Eye

"Red eye," as it is commonly called, is an infection of the superficial cells of the eye.

SIGNS AND SYMPTOMS:
1. Redness
2. Itching
3. Pus or watery discharge from the inner corner of the eye
4. Severe eye pain is not usually present.

TREATMENT:

1. Cool compresses applied to the eye four times a day
2. Medication—an antibiotic eyedrop may be used; Neosporin or Sulamyd 10% ophthalmic drops should be administered every 2–3 hours for at least 3 days.

Note: Severe eye pain may be caused by a tiny foreign object embedded on the surface of the eye or eyelid (see section 4.4, "Eye Injuries"), or a superficial scratch of the cornea. Treatment is to flush the eye with sterile water or Dacriose irrigating solution, administer an antibiotic eyedrop as mentioned above, and put a patch over the eye.

3.2b Ear

1. External Ear Infection, or "Swimmer's Ear"

SIGNS AND SYMPTOMS:

Itching, pain (may be severe); scaling of ear canal skin may be present.

TREATMENT:

1. Instill Auralgan or Cortisporin eardrops, 2 drops, 4 times a day, into the affected ear.
2. Place an earwick (a piece of cotton saturated with alcohol) into the external ear canal 3 times a day.
3. Administer pain medication if necessary, such as Tylenol #3, orally, one every 4 hours.
4. Although the treatment is controversial, ampicillin or erythromycin may be administered orally, 250 mg every 6 hours.

PREVENTION:

Persons prone to swimmer's ear should put several drops of alcohol in the ears after swimming and dry off as soon as possible.

2. Middle Ear Infection: Otitis Media

SIGNS AND SYMPTOMS:
1. Pain in the affected ear
2. Fever and/or chills
3. A feeling of fullness in the ear

TREATMENT:
1. Administer antibiotics: penicillin, ampicillin, erythromycin, or Keflex. Dosage: 250 mg every 6 hours for 10 days.
2. Pain medication such as Tylenol #3, as needed.
3. A decongestant may be helpful, such as Sudafed, 60 mg orally, 3 times a day.
4. A heating pad applied to the ear may help control pain.

3.2c Tonsillitis and Strep Throat

SYMPTOMS:
1. Sore throat
2. Fever and/or chills
3. Headache; malaise
4. Tonsils red and swollen. Pus is usually present.

TREATMENT:
1. Bed rest
2. Encourage oral fluid intake.
3. Decongestant may be helpful, such as Sudafed, 60 mg 3 times a day.

4. Antibiotics, such as penicillin, ampicillin, erythromycin, or Keflex, 250 mg every 6 hours, orally, for 10 days.
5. Saltwater gargle (½ teaspoon salt in ½ glass of water) every 2–3 hours.
6. Pain medication, such as Tylenol #3 orally, or, if swallowing is too painful, Demerol, 50–75 mg IM.

3.3 Respiratory Infections

3.3a Cold or Flu

SYMPTOMS:

1. General malaise
2. Sore throat, runny nose
3. Fever may or may not be present.

TREATMENT:

1. Rest, drink clear liquids, and increase vitamin intake (multipurpose vitamin and 1–2 gm vitamin C).
2. Administer aspirin or Tylenol, one or 2 tablets every 4 hours, to get fever down to 101 degrees orally.
3. Administer a decongestant such as Sudafed, if needed, 60 mg 3 times a day.
4. Antibiotics generally are not needed.

Why Antibiotics and Flu Shots Won't Help a Cold

Different germs cause different diseases. Viruses, for example, cause poliomyelitis, viral pneumonitis, and influenza ("flu"). Another type of germ, the bacterium, causes strep throat, gonorrhea, rheumatic fever, and staphylococcal infections.

In order to cure a disease, it's necessary to eliminate the germ causing it. You can do that by taking medicine (pills, shots) or by allowing the body's own natural defense mechanisms to destroy the germ.

If a medicine has not been developed that can kill a certain germ, you have to follow the latter course: Allow the body to rest, and relieve symptoms until the disease naturally runs its course.

Antibiotics kill or arrest the growth of bacteria, but they have little or no effect on viruses. Consequently, they are generally only effective against a bacterially induced illness.

The flu shot is a vaccine, which means it contains a weakened version of the organism that could infect you should you be exposed to it—in this case the influenza virus. If you have a flu shot, you will be partially or completely immune to the influenza virus, but you will have no protection against the viruses that cause the common cold.

No medicine yet exists that will kill or stop the growth of common cold viruses. The only way to rid yourself of a cold is to allow your body to overcome the virus in its own way. You can take aspirin for your aches, pains, and fever; cough remedies; and preparations that will dry up your runny nose; but you can't take any medicine that will cure your cold. If you have adequate rest and drink plenty of fluids, your cold will usually be gone in 5–7 days.

Another reason not to take antibiotics unnecessarily is that antibiotics don't know the difference between harmful and nonharmful bacteria. Your body contains both kinds, and the nonharmful ones keep harmful organisms under control. Antibiotics kill all bacteria, and can permit other illnesses or side effects to occur. Candidiasis, an uncomfortable vaginal itch and discharge, is one consequence of antibiotic therapy; diarrhea is another.

3.3b Upper Respiratory Infection (URI)

Upper respiratory infection is usually caused by a virus. Again, there are no medications that can kill the virus germs that cause influenza, colds, and many other upper respiratory infections. Only bacterial organisms can be killed with antibiotics such as penicillin. Any respiratory infection is more or less contagious, so don't share spoons, cups, or kisses until the patient is well.

TREATMENT:

1. Keep warm, and rest as much as possible.
2. Encourage consumption of fluids; solid foods are not that important, as appetite will return when the patient is well.
3. If temperature goes over 101 degress orally, aspirin or Tylenol may be administered (see section 3.1).
4. If nausea and vomiting are present, restrict diet to clear liquids, juices, and soups. Small amounts of liquids taken often will stay down better than a large amount taken at once. Fluids taken by the patient must be enough to keep up with fluid loss due to sweating, vomiting, diarrhea, and fever.
5. If a high temperature is present (over 101 degrees orally), and does not come down despite proper doses of aspirin or Tylenol, begin bathing the patient in lukewarm or cool water until the temperature falls to the 101-degree range. The water should not be so cold as to cause shivering (see section 3.1). Avoid excitement. Use only light covers and clothing so that body heat can escape.

6. If the throat is sore, have the patient gargle with saltwater (½ teaspoon of salt in ½ glass of water). Try cool or cold packs on the outside of the throat for comfort.
7. If the nose or throat is dry, encourage still more fluids and add humidity to the air with pans of evaporating water on the galley stove, or with a steaming tub or shower, if available.
8. If cough is present, have patient drink lots of fluids to moisten and loosen sticky mucus. Non-prescription cough medicines containing an expectorant, such as Robitussin, also help to moisten mucus.
9. If there is croup (croupy coughing sounds like the braying of a donkey) or if breathing is difficult, have the patient breathe steam for a few minutes, then wrap the patient in blankets and take on deck to breathe colder air. The patient can also breathe over a bucket with ice in it. Many times, this will help alleviate the bronchospasm that causes croupy breathing.

IF THE PATIENT GETS WORSE

The patient with a minor respiratory infection may get pneumonia, an ear infection, or other illness. If the condition gets worse instead of better, especially if you notice any of the following symptoms, administer antibiotics as directed in section 3.3c.

SYMPTOMS:

1. A very high temperature, in spite of measures taken to lower the fever
2. Bloody sputum or chest pain
3. Difficulty in breathing, especially if it's getting worse

4. Skin, lips, or fingernail bed color change from pink to light gray or bluish color
5. Stiffness that prevents bending the neck (cannot put chin on chest without severe pain or headache)
6. Thick yellow or greenish drainage from the ears or sinuses

3.3c Pneumonia

Pneumonia can be caused by many different types of infectious organisms. We'll briefly discuss two main groups: bacterial and viral. Often, the symptoms of each are hard to differentiate without laboratory facilities, as there is a great deal of overlap. Therefore, the following is a very general outline, but may be useful to you in determining whether to administer an antibiotic. Otherwise, the treatment remains similar for either kind.

1. Bacterial

SIGNS AND SYMPTOMS:

a. Fever
b. Cough
c. Patient will usually be coughing up greenish-yellow phlegm.
d. Increased difficulty breathing

TREATMENT:

a. Begin an antibiotic, such as penicillin, ampicillin, erythromycin, or Keflex, dosage of 250 mg every 6 hours, orally. If patient is unable to tolerate oral fluids or antibiotics due to vomiting, penicillin, 300,000–600,000 units IM, may be administered. See "Procedures," sections 15.1, 15.2, and 15.3.

2. *Viral*

SIGNS AND SYMPTOMS:

    a. Often imitate flu or common cold symptoms
    b. Fatigue
    c. Headache
    d. Muscle aches
    e. Cough with little or no sputum production

TREATMENT:

    a. In general, an antibiotic is not indicated for a viral pneumonia. However, if the sick crew member is getting worse day by day, and medical assistance is not available soon, then a 10-day course of antibiotics such as erythromycin or tetracycline, 250 mg every 6 hours, is probably justified to prevent additional infection from a bacterial source.
    b. See treatment of fever, section 3.1.
    c. Encourage adequate oral fluid intake.

3.4 *Genitourinary Infections*

3.4a *Urinary Tract Infections*

SIGNS AND SYMPTOMS:

    1. Chills and/or fever
    2. Pain or burning on urination
    3. Pain in the lower back or flank
    4. Passing blood in the urine
    5. Increased urge to urinate, with little actual passage of urine

TREATMENT:

1. Encourage a large increase in fluid intake. Restrict the use of alcoholic beverages.
2. Administer antibiotics, any of the following:
   a. Ampicillin, 250 mg every 6 hours for 10 days
   b. Azogantrisin, 4 immediately, then 2, 4 times a day for 10 days.
   c. Septra, 2 twice a day for 10 days.
   d. If the inability to urinate continues well past 8 hours, the severe discomfort may require passing a urethral catheter into the bladder to allow drainage of urine. A Foley catheter should be used and left in place. See "Procedures," section 15.7—Bladder Catheterization.

1. Epididymitis

This is an inflammation of one of the spermatic cord structures of the testes.

SIGNS AND SYMPTOMS:

1. The testicle on the involved side will appear swollen, red, warm, and cordlike to the touch, and will be very sensitive to pressure.
2. Elevated temperature

TREATMENT:

1. Administer antibiotics, such as:
   a. Ampicillin, 250 mg every 6 hours for 10 days
   b. Septra, 2 every 12 hours for 10 days
2. Wear an athletic supporter
3. Bed rest

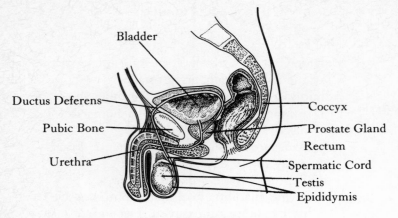

Bladder

Ductus Deferens

Pubic Bone

Urethra

Coccyx

Prostate Gland

Rectum

Spermatic Cord

Testis

Epididymis

Male genitourinary system

3.4b Sexually Transmitted Diseases

1. Gonorrhea

SIGNS AND SYMPTOMS:

1. Men: Milky white to yellowish-red discharge from the urethra (end of the penis), associated with burning and pain on urination
2. Women: Often without symptoms; may have had contact with a known male carrier

TREATMENT:

1. Tetracycline orally, 500 mg every 6 hours for 10 days, *or*
2. Ampicillin orally, single dose of 3.5 grams (this would be seven 500-mg or fourteen 250-mg tablets or capsules, all at once). As this is such a large dose, take on a full stomach to prevent nausea.

Note: As the organism responsible for gonorrhea becomes more resistant to the antibiotics now used, more and more treatment failures are being seen. Should a urethral discharge continue, other venereal organisms may be responsible, and a continued regime of tetracycline, 500 mg every 6 hours, is recommended.

2. Syphilis

Syphilis is referred to as "the great masquerader," because it mimics so many other diseases with so many clinical symptoms.

SIGNS AND SYMPTOMS:

Primary syphilis:
   a. Skin lesion, called a "chancre," which is a painless, ulcerated area with raised borders; variable in size, but can be up to the size of a 25-cent piece.
   b. Multiple lesions may occur; most are on the genitalia, but can be found on the lips, or any other part of the body.

Secondary syphilis:
   a. Various skin rashes and mucus membrane lesions occur, about two months after the primary chancre. The rash does not itch, and may be localized to the palms of the hands or the soles of the feet.

TREATMENT:
   a. Tetracycline, 500 mg orally, every 6 hours for 15 days.
   b. If available, give an IM injection of benzathine penicillin G, 2.4 million units in a single dose.

3. Herpes Simplex

Genital herpes is estimated to have infected over 20 million people in the United States. The disease-causing agent is a virus, the Herpes Simplex Virus (HSV), of which there are two types. HSV-1 is the type associated with cold sores on the lips. Almost everyone who periodically develops cold sores on their lips has the HSV-1. Genital herpes infections, on the other hand, are most often caused by the HSV-2 and are usually associated with symptoms, especially during the first infection.

SIGNS AND SYMPTOMS (of first, or primary infection):

1. One or more lesions (at the site of contact) on the genitals. Herpes lesions begin as blisters, which rupture in a few days and develop into ulcers, small depressions, or craters in the skin. The lesions usually last from 2–6 weeks. The virus is present in the herpes lesion, and can be transmitted to other people by sexual activity. Due to the detection of the HSV-1 on genitalia and the HSV-2 on lips, oral sex has been implicated in the transmission and reversal of sites of the infection of the virus types.
2. Pain associated with the lesions, especially with urination. The primary infection is usually always the worst in terms of local discomfort at the site of the lesions.
3. Burning and itching of the lesions
4. General feeling of malaise (aches and pains)
5. The vast majority of herpes infections involve just the symptoms and lesions in the genital area. Herpes is not felt to lead to sterility.
6. Occasionally, fever, neck pain, and photophobia (sensitivity to light) will develop. If these symp-

toms occur, medical assistance should be obtained, as these may indicate neurological involvement.

SIGNS AND SYMPTOMS (of recurrent infections):

1. Lesions similar to ones in initial infection, but of shorter duration, usually lasting 2–10 days
2. Pain, itching, and burning at the site of the lesions, but less severe than in the initial infection

TREATMENT:

Currently, there is no known cure for herpes infections of either type. As the virus is present in the lesions, sexual relations should be avoided while the lesions are present. Although it has not yet been proven, the use of a condom during sexual activity may aid in decreasing the transmission of the disease.

Recently, a drug called Zovirax (acyclovir) ointment 5% has been used to treat the initial onset of genital herpes. A decrease in the associated pain in the area and a decrease in the healing time of the lesions have been demonstrated. The ointment is applied to lesions 6 times a day for 7 days. It does not prevent recurrence, nor has it been tested for use in pregnant women.

Note: Sitting in a warm bath, if one is available, 3–5 times a day, will keep the inflamed areas clean and help relieve pain and discomfort. Keep the lesions as dry as possible between baths. Since the lesions will go away without any scarring, treatment is directed at reducing pain and minimizing the danger of infecting the ulcerated areas with bacteria.

3.5 Skin Infections

3.5a Saltwater boils (the bane of the offshore sailor)

TREATMENT:

1. Follow directions for the treatment of simple wound infections, section 3.5b. Usually, a topical antibiotic cream or ointment will not get rid of these areas.
2. Incision and drainage may be necessary if the boil is large enough, is "pointing," and is not draining the pus spontaneously.
   a. Gently cleanse the area with betadine.
   b. Using a sterile scalpel blade, prick the skin for ¼–½ inch across the boil and allow the pus to drain from the area.
   c. Apply warm compresses to the area for 20 minutes, 4 times a day.
   d. Cover the area with sterile dressing, if possible.
   e. Try to keep dry (Good luck!) as saltwater is a skin irritant.

3.5b Wound Infections

Simple wound infections can easily ruin an otherwise uneventful voyage. More serious infections may even become life-threatening if left untreated.

SIGNS AND SYMPTOMS (of simple wound infections):

1. Redness, swelling, and warmth around the wound site
2. There may be red streaks around the wound site.
3. Pus may be draining from the area.
4. Fever and/or chills may be present.

34

TREATMENT:

1. Apply warm Epsom-salts compresses to the area. Leave on for 10–15 minutes, 3–4 times a day.
2. A topical antibiotic cream or ointment such as Polymyxin or neosporin may be applied to the area after the warm compresses.
3. Administer antibiotics orally, such as ampicillin, erythromycin, or Keflex, 250 mg every six hours for 7–10 days.

3.5c Fungal Infections

In general, try to keep the skin surfaces cool and dry. Towel off perspiration after exercise. Don't go around in bare feet; wear shoes.

SYMPTOMS AND TREATMENT OF COMMON FUNGAL PROBLEMS:

1. Ringworm (of body or scalp)
   Symptoms: Slight itching, and a reddish-gray, round, bald lesion
   Treatment: Griseofulvin, orally, 0.25 mg twice a day for 14 days.
2. Jock Itch
   Symptoms: Marked itching of the groin, redness of the inner thighs or perineal region
   Treatment: Tinactin solution or cream applied to the area 3–4 times a day; or Monistat-Derm applied twice a day for at least 14 days
3. Athlete's Foot
   Symptoms: Itching and stinging of the area between the toes; may involve the soles of the feet; skin may be cracked, and red, sore spots may be present.
   Treatment: Same as that for #2 above, applied for 30 days.

4. Eye, Ear, and Nose Problems

4.1 Nosebleed

Bleeding is usually caused by a tiny split in the mucosa, which lines the inside of the nose. It usually takes 8–10 days for complete healing to occur; until then, be very careful not to dislodge the clot or scab sealing the bleeding site.

TREATMENT:
1. If spotty bleeding occurs, simply rest and wait for it to stop. Avoid hot foods, as the heat or steam may dilate the nasal blood vessels and cause further bleeding.
2. If bleeding becomes moderate or heavy, put a piece of cotton into the nose and pinch the nose gently but firmly, holding the whole nose and pressing both sides against the middle part. If this controls the bleeding, hold the pressure for at least 5 minutes. If bleeding starts again when the pressure is released, blow out all the clots and repeat pinching for 10–15 more minutes.
3. An oral pain medication, such as Tylenol #3, may be given if necessary. Avoid aspirin or any medication that contains aspirin, as it will affect the body's clotting mechanisms.
4. If these measures do not work, and bleeding continues unabated, the bleeding may be coming from a site very high in the nose. In this case,

packing the nose with a Foley catheter is the simplest treatment.

a. Place the patient in an upright, sitting position.

b. Administer a pain medication if one has not already been given. Tylenol #3 will suffice. A sedative, such as Valium, 5 mg orally, may be given instead. The patient should be well-sedated but conscious, because the procedure and the result are both uncomfortable.

c. Lubricate with Vaseline a Foley catheter with a 10-cc balloon on the end.

d. Insert the catheter into the bleeding nostril, along the floor of the nose, until resistance stops. The tip of the catheter is now in the nasopharynx, and passing the catheter further might cause choking and gagging. Stop there.

e. Inject 5–7 cc of air into the balloon portal (this will be diagrammed in the Foley package), then pull the catheter back toward you, exerting firm but gentle traction.

f. Without letting go of the traction, tape the end of the catheter you are holding to the patient's forehead. The catheter may be left in place for 12–24 hours.

g. To remove, deflate the balloon by drawing the air out of the portal with the empty syringe and needle.

h. Wait 15 minutes or so to see if the bleeding resumes. It it does, reinflate the balloon and leave the catheter in for another 12 hours. If bleeding does not resume, slowly pull on the catheter to remove it.

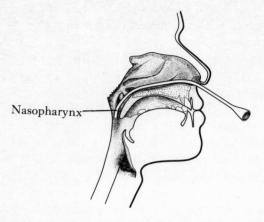

Nosebleed—after the balloon is blown up, gentle traction on the catheter is maintained so that the balloon occludes the bleeding site at the rear of the nares.

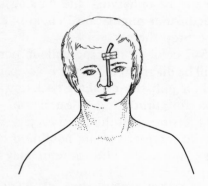

The catheter is then taped to the forehead.

5. To Prevent Reoccurrence:
    a. Do not pick, twist, dab, or otherwise handle the nose.
    b. Blow only gently, and as little as possible. Soften the mucosa before blowing with a

little water sniffed or dropped into the nose.

c. Avoid deep bending, and other positions in which the head is lowered far down. Rest and sleep with the head slightly elevated.

d. Avoid heavy lifting and straining.

e. Drink plenty of fluids, especially when the weather is dry.

4.2 Barotrauma (Ruptured Eardrum)

In snorkeling or diving, if you are unable to clear your eustachian tubes (they teach you how to do this in scuba lessons), the eardrum, or typanic membrane, may rupture. This is because the eustachian tube connects the middle ear to the throat and equalizes the air pressure between those areas. If this pressure is unequal, and yawning or swallowing doesn't open up the eustachian tube, the pressure buildup may be severe enough to cause the eardrum to rupture.

SIGNS AND SYMPTOMS:

1. Severe pain
2. Loss of hearing
3. Dizziness
4. Bleeding from ear

TREATMENT:

1. Place a piece of sterile cotton in the ear. Do *not* use eardrops or wash the ear with water or oil.
2. Administer an antibiotic, such as penicillin or Keflex, 250 mg 4 times a day.

3. Administer pain medication if needed, such as Tylenol #3, orally, 1 every 4 hours.
4. Encourage the patient to rest.
5. Decongestant may be helpful; Sudafed 60 mg, orally 3 times a day, or Afrin nasal spray, 2 inhalations 4 times a day.

4.3 Foreign Object in the Ear

Usually, the foreign object is some kind of insect. If a bug decides to use your ear as a home, use mineral oil or oily ear drops to drown it. A small pair of forceps can be used to grasp and gently remove it.

4.4 Eye Injuries

For nonpenetrating injuries involving minute foreign particles (such as dust), corrosives (such as battery acid), or chemicals, the following generalized treatment will suffice.

TREATMENT:

1. Flush the eye with clean water for at least 20 minutes. Seawater can be used if necessary.
2. Place a patch over the closed eye and instruct the patient to rest.
3. If infection occurs, see section 3.2a.

For a foreign object embedded on the inner surface of the eyelid, or on the superficial surface of the eye itself, gently try to remove it with a sterile cotton-tipped swab. It's sometimes possible to use the tip of a sterile 25-gauge needle to pry the foreign object off the surface of the eye. Obviously, this will not be easy to do aboard a vessel. If you attempt it, do so very gently and slowly, and do *not* dig, poke, or continuously scrape the surface of the eye. If you cannot remove the foreign body, instill several drops of an antibiotic solution, such as Sulamyd 10% ophthalmic solution, and patch the eye, as medical assistance of some kind will be necessary.

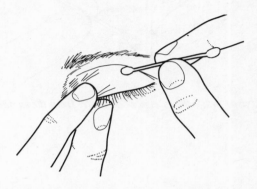

Invert the upper lid with gentle traction on the eyelashes, using a Q-Tip for leverage. Flip the lower border of the lid over the Q-Tip.

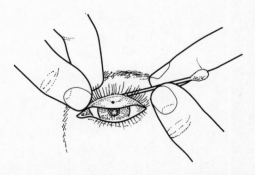

Here, the lid is inverted. Note the foreign body on the surface of the upper lid.

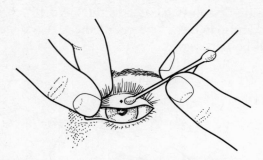

A Q-Tip is used to lift the foreign body gently from the surface of the lid.

5. Abdominal Pain

5.1 Generalities

At sea, abdominal pain can result from seasickness, tension, fatigue, or poor diet. Once these potential causes have been ruled out, abdominal pain becomes one of the more difficult medical symptoms to evaluate. It can occur when various organs (such as the stomach, duodenum, gallbladder, intestines, appendix, etc.) are not functioning properly.

In order to determine the exact area of the pain, and relate that to what may be the cause of the patient's distress, find out the following:

1. Where did the pain first begin? Does the pain stay in one place or move around to other areas?
2. How long has the pain been there? Has it gotten somewhat better, only to worsen? Or has it been very severe from its onset?
3. Has there been any nausea or vomiting? If so, how many times, and what did the vomitus contain—foodstuff, bright red blood, dark coffee ground–like material, mucus?
4. Does the patient have a fever? If so, how high is it? Are there chills present?
5. Has there been any previous episode of a similar kind of pain? If so, what was the cause and how was the pain treated?
6. Does anything the patient does make the pain feel better or worse?

At this point, you will have several answers and probably no diagnosis. Evaluating these answers will be a matter of forming a differential diagnosis and proceeding with an organized treatment plan.

The following guidelines can be used until you reach a more exact diagnosis:

1. No solid foods, no alcoholic beverages. Small sips of water may be given.
2. If pain is intense, administer a pain medication, such as Demerol, 50 mg IM. Morphine, 4–8 mg IM, can be used instead. See Appendix 2, "Adult Dosages of Common Medications," for precautions in the use of these potent narcotic medications.
3. If nausea or vomiting is present, administer an antiemetic such as Tigan, 2 cc IM, or Compazine, 10 mg IM. See directions for giving IM injections under "Procedures," section 15.3.
4. An enema may be given, but *only* if appendicitis has been ruled out. A prepackaged enema like the Fleet or a home-style one may be given. Give only one enema; do not repeat.
5. Record urine output, noting the number of cc's per hour. One measuring cup = 8 oz = 240 cc's (or milliliters); ½ cup = 120 cc's, etc.
6. If the patient's temperature is over 101 degrees orally, administer broad-spectrum antibiotics, such as ampicillin or erythromycin, 250 mg every 6 hours, orally.
7. If there is no improvement, and the vomiting is getting worse, a nasogastric tube may have to be inserted to evacuate the stomach contents and provide relief of gastric spasm. This is not an innocuous procedure; see directions on how to

pass a nasogastric tube under "Procedures," section 15.5.

Note: It should be emphasized that the treatment of abdominal pain aboard a boat should be aimed not just at improving a patient's symptoms, but perhaps at keeping the patient alive until definitive medical treatment can be obtained.

5.2 Seasickness

SYMPTOMS:

Fatigue, lethargy, drowsiness, stomach-awareness, nausea, pallor of face, cold sweat, headache, belching. These may lead to vomiting.

HOW AND WHY:

The theory goes something like this: various receptors in the brain control balance, movement, and awareness of where you are relative to other objects. On land, these receptors anticipate sensory signals and allow the body to move relative to the prediction of signals (what the brain *thinks* will happen) and the signals as they are received (what *actually* happens). When continuous disturbances of balance, movement, and awareness occur, as they can aboard any boat, "sensory conflict" increases, and a physiologic signal is sent to the brain that activates a vomiting reflex.

WHAT TO DO ABOUT IT:

1. Stay in the area of the vessel which has the least motion (usually amidships or slightly aft).
2. Go on deck and look around at the horizon and at any distant objects in view.
3. Keep occupied and try to think about other things.
4. Go below only for short periods of time if you're feeling sick.

45

5. Try to restrain your movements and actions. If you must move around deck, wear a safety harness.
6. Get adequate rest and sleep as much as possible. This decreases sensory conflict.
7. Drink fluids. This is especially important during the first 12 hours of a voyage; after that, adequate fluids and salt intake should be maintained. Have tea, Jell-O, soft drinks, and broth. Avoid heavy meals that could promote nausea and vomiting. In the second 12 hours, add soup, applesauce, bananas, crackers, and toast with jelly.
8. Avoid alcoholic beverages, as these affect the brain as well as the balance mechanism of the body.
9. Although I haven't tried these myself, friends tell me that drinking a few drops of aromatic bitters, or taking a teaspoonful or so of ginger root will calm the stomach. Acupressure is also said to help; apply pressure to the inner forearm, three fingerbreadths above the wrist joint and in between the two flexor tendons going to the fingers. Good luck!

MEDICATIONS:

There are a number of medications for motion sickness, such as Dramamine, Bonine, and Compazine. See dosages in Appendix 2.

A newer drug, which I have prescribed with good results, is Transderm-Scōp, a stick-on button placed behind the ear. The drug is absorbed through the skin into the bloodstream, giving the patient a three-day source of medication. It should *not* be used by pregnant women or people with glaucoma, peptic ulcers, or bladder obstruction. Side effects in some people include dry mouth and drowsiness.

Note: One of the principal side effects of these drugs is fatigue. Beware of the crew member on watch who has taken any sort of medication; falling asleep at the helm may occur.

Note: No matter which medication a crew member chooses to take, he or she should take it *before* severe seasickness occurs.

5.3 Constipation

Lack of regular bowel movements is one of the most common ailments on any voyage. This is frequently a result of physical inactivity, inadequate fluids, or a change in the daily routine from landbound to seagoing life, and most people will encounter constipation at one time or another. Care should be taken on a long voyage to note the frequency of bowel movements for all crew members (Yes, I know this is compulsive behavior on the part of the captain . . .) Depending on the individual's metabolism, if two days go by without a bowel movement, treatment should be initiated.

TREATMENT:

1. Watch your diet. Avoid heavy, constipating foods like rice, bananas, and starches. Eat stewed or raw vegetables and fruits, especially prunes; high-fiber cereals; and fluids.
2. Most cases of constipation can be treated with the above dietary modifications. However, laxatives (not to be used daily) may be helpful. Mineral oil, Metamucil, Milk of Magnesia, or a Fleet enema may be used.

5.4 Diarrhea

There are multiple causes of diarrhea, but it is easiest to consider treatment if we classify the causes into two main subgroups:

1. Simple, uncomplicated diarrhea, associated with mild infection, but no signs of shock.
2. Severe diarrhea, complicated by more severe infection, which may lead to shock secondary to loss of fluids and electrolytes.

Examples of Type 1:
a. *Traveler's diarrhea* ("turista")—no mucus or blood in stool; abdominal cramps; frequent diarrhea.
b. *Acute gastroenteritis*—acute abdominal pains which are colicky (intermittent); possible chills and fever; explosive diarrhea; no mucus or blood in stool.

TREATMENT:
1. Fluid intake must be maintained. See treatment for seasickness.
2. Encourage rest.
3. Although the following may be used to ease symptoms, doctors disagree on whether they do more harm than good:
    a. Lomotil tablets: 2 tablets immediately, followed by one tablet after each loose stool, to a maximum of 8 tablets a day.
    b. Imodium capsules: 2 capsules after each unformed stool, to a total of 8 capsules a day.
    c. Kaopectate: 4–8 tablespoons up to 4 times a day.
    d. Pepto-Bismol (a bismuth compound): 2 oz

every hour up to 8 doses to reduce diarrhea; 1–2 oz 4 times a day as preventive treatment.

Examples of Type 2:
a. *Giardiasis*—Infection by the Giardia lamblia organism. Usually contracted by drinking contaminated water. If contamination is suspected, boil all water before using. Drink bottled beverages if possible. Consider this situation as infectious to all crew members, and observe sanitary conditions to minimize the spread of infection.

SIGNS AND SYMPTOMS:
1. Severe abdominal cramps
2. Explosive, watery stools which are foul-smelling
3. Muscle aches and pains; weight loss

TREATMENT:

Flagyl, 250 mg orally, 3 times a day for 7 days. (*Note:* At present, this mode of treatment is being reviewed for approval by the Food and Drug Administration.)

b. *Shigellosis* (dysentery)—This is similar to acute gastroenteritis, but more severe.

SIGNS AND SYMPTOMS:
1. Abdominal cramps with frequent watery diarrhea
2. Fever and/or chills
3. Blood, mucus, and/or pus in stool
4. Possible nausea or vomiting

TREATMENT:
1. Bed rest
2. Encourage consumption of oral fluids.

3. Intravenous fluids, if necessary (see "Procedures," 15.1 and 15.2)
4. *Avoid* Lomotil, Imodium, Kaopectate.
5. Administer Septra, 2 tablets twice a day for 5 days, or ampicillin, 250 mg four times a day for 5 days.

c. *Campylobacter*—This is becoming known as one of the most frequent causes of acute diarrhea in the world.

SIGNS AND SYMPTOMS:
1. Acute onset
2. Fever
3. Blood in stool
4. Abdominal pain
5. Nausea and vomiting

TREATMENT:

Erythromycin, 500 mg 4 times a day orally for 10 days.

Note: If food poisoning is the suspected cause of abdominal pain, see under the heading "Poisoning," section 11.5.

5.5 *Ulcer*

In the patient with a history of ulcer, or of taking antacids and/or eating a special bland diet over a long period of time, severe abdominal pain may be secondary to a perforated ulcer or GI (gastrointestinal) hemorrhage. For these patients, treatment is aimed at getting past the life-threatening crisis.

SIGNS AND SYMPTOMS:
1. A burning, cramplike aching pain in the center or upper abdomen. Usually, the pain occurs 45–

60 minutes after meals, and may worsen between midnight and 2 A.M. Pain is relieved by
food, milk, or antacids.
2. Nausea and vomiting may be present.
3. In a GI hemorrhage, onset is typified by weakness, faintness, cool, moist skin, and vomiting
coffee ground–like material or bright red blood,
or the passage of dark, tarry stools.
4. In a perforated ulcer, which usually occurs in
males between the ages of 25 and 45 years, the
onset of pain is acute and located in the upper
abdomen. The pain may radiate to the shoulder or to the right lower quadrant. It is associated with nausea, vomiting, fever, increased
pulse rate, and rigid abdominal wall muscles.
The patient's belly will feel stiff as a plank to
touch.

TREATMENT:
1. Immediately put the patient to rest.
2. Administer pain medication, such as Demerol,
50–75 mg IM.
3. Withhold all food and drink; the patient should
take nothing by mouth.
4. Pass a nasogastric (NG) tube into the stomach
to allow the stomach contents to drain. (See
"Procedures," section 15.5.)
5. Administer an antacid, such as Maalox, through
the NG tube, one teaspoon every 1–2 hours.
6. Administer an antibiotic, such as penicillin,
600,000 units, every 6 hours IM, for a minimum
of 3 days.
7. Keep a record of urine output.
8. Keep a record of the patient's temperature.
9. Administer fluids, either through the NG tube

at a rate of several ounces every few hours, or begin an intravenous (IV) infusion and give fluids as directed in "Procedures," sections 15.1 and 15.2.

With the above treatment, improvement should be noted in 7–10 days. Pain and nausea should be gone, temperature should fall to normal, and the abdomen should not be tender to the touch. At this time, stop all medication. Start sipping water. If no nausea or bellyache returns, remove the NG tube and gradually give the patient a soft, bland diet, as well as antacids, 1–2 teaspoonsful every hour. At this dosage, antacids can be constipating, so a laxative may also be needed.

AFTERCARE:

1. Give no alcohol, spicy food, caffeine-containing beverages, or known irritant.
2. Use an antacid, such as Maalox, on a regular basis.
3. Avoid stress; solve problems as quickly as possible.
4. Avoid aspirin, as it may irritate the stomach lining; use Tylenol (acetaminophen) if needed.

5.6 Appendicitis

SIGNS AND SYMPTOMS:

1. Pain, beginning in the upper to midabdominal area or around the navel, then shifting to the right-lower quadrant of the abdomen
2. Nausea and vomiting
3. An unwillingness to eat
4. Constipation may occur, as the patient will be

unwilling to go to the head because bearing down increases the abdominal pain.

5. Gentle touching of the right-lower quadrant will cause localized pain in that area. The pain will become worse when the patient coughs.

TREATMENT:

1. Bed rest
2. Give the patient nothing by mouth.
3. Administer pain medication, such as Demerol, 50–75 mg IM.
4. Administer medication to control nausea and vomiting, such as Tigan, 2 cc IM, or Compazine, 10 mg IM.
5. Do *not* give an enema.
6. If the patient has severe, unrelenting pain associated with nausea and vomiting, administer an antibiotic, such as penicillin, 600,000 units IM.
7. With recovery:
   a. Give the patient only clear fluids to soft solids for 4–5 days.
   b. A mild laxative may be administered if needed; do *not* use an enema.
   c. Continue antibiotics orally for 7–10 days (if antibiotics have been used); penicillin, ampicillin, or Keflex, 250–500 mg every 6 hours.
8. If the pain worsens, or the patient does not improve, a burst appendix may be indicated. Further medical treatment is mandatory, and is beyond the scope of this text, since surgery will probably have to be performed.

5.7 Hernia

In males, a hernia is a weakness in some of the muscle fiber groups of the inguinal canal, which may result in protrusion of the intestine into the scrotal sac, thereby causing lower abdominal and scrotal pain.

SIGNS AND SYMPTOMS:

1. Lower abdominal or scrotal pain
2. Localized swelling in the above areas

TREATMENT:

1. Position the patient lying on his back with his knees bent up.
2. Lift the scrotal sac and gently allow the intestine to move back through the inguinal ring.
3. Patient should wear a good athletic supporter and avoid all heavy lifting.
4. If the hernia (or "rupture") does not reduce with this treatment, keep the patient lying flat. Administer pain medication, such as Demerol, 50–75 mg, IM, and seek medical assistance as soon as possible.

5.8 Kidney Stone

A kidney stone can form anywhere in the urinary tract; that is, the kidney, ureter, or bladder. Stones are made of calcium or uric acid crystals.

SIGNS AND SYMPTOMS:

1. Severe pain of sudden onset, located in the low back and radiating around the side into the lower abdomen, and into the testicle in males, or the bladder area in females.

2. The pain may come and go, but is severe when it returns.
3. Nausea and vomiting may occur, along with sweating and anxiety.
4. There may be an urge to urinate, although little urine may be able to be passed.
5. A visible reddish color to the urine may be observed; this is blood being passed. At times, frank, bright red blood is passed.

TREATMENT:

1. Administer pain medication, such as Demerol, 75 mg IM.
2. Administer medication for nausea and vomiting if needed: Tigan, 2 cc, or Compazine, 10 mg IM.
3. Oral fluids should be encouraged as soon as possible. This is very important, as it helps "flush" the urinary tract and allows small stones to pass more easily. Fluid intake should be 2000–3000 cc (2–3 quarts) per day. If vomiting prevents oral intake, intravenous fluids should be administered; see "Procedures," sections 1 and 2.
4. Administer antibiotics, orally if possible. The choice is wide: ampicillin, 250 mg every 6 hours, Septra, 2 tablets every 12 hours, or Gantrisin, 4 immediately, followed by 2 tablets 4 times a day. Whichever antibiotic is used, continue it for a 10-day period.
5. Foods to *avoid:* caffeine-containing beverages, alcoholic beverages, certain fruits such as apples or grapes.

6. Heart Attack

A heart attack or "coronary" signifies that the blood supply to one or more of the blood vessels to the heart has been disrupted. Heart attack may lead to unconsciousness or complete collapse (cardiovascular shock). The signs and symptoms of a heart attack may be variable; the following are some of the more common complaints:

SIGNS AND SYMPTOMS:
1. Chest pain. This is probably the first and most common symptom. The pain may be crushing, a dull ache, or a pressure sensation over the chest. The pain may radiate into the neck, chin, shoulders, or down one or both arms; one or both hands may be numb.
2. Apprehension
3. Shortness of breath
4. Nausea and vomiting
5. Sweating
6. Vague feeling of indigestion

TREATMENT:
1. Cardiopulmonary resuscitation (CPR) if necessary; see section 2.1. Otherwise, see below.
2. Put the victim in a sitting position and loosen clothing.
3. Give nitroglycerin, $1/150$ grain; place one tablet under the tongue where it will dissolve; this may be repeated every 5–10 minutes 2 times more

56

for a total of 3 tablets. Nitroglycerin is a very potent vasodilator, used to increase the blood supply to the heart vessels.

4. Administer pain medication: Demerol, 50–100 mg IM. Morphine, 4–8 mg IM, may be given instead, if available.
5. Encourage quiet rest; do not allow the patient to move around.
6. Seek medical facilities as soon as possible.

7. Unconsciousness

7.1 Generalities

Unconsciousness or coma is not a disease; it is usually the result of an injury or illness. Although we should make every attempt to diagnose the cause of unconsciousness, the treatment principles remain unchanged. Indeed, as you will see below, it does no good to know a diagnosis if the victim isn't getting enough air to his heart, lungs, brain, and kidneys; or aspirates vomit in his airway. No matter what the cause, the following guidelines should be observed:

TREATMENT:

1. Is the person breathing? If not, begin CPR; see section 2.1.
2. Is there a good pulse and heartbeat? If not, begin CPR.
3. Are the skin, lips, and tongue pink? If blue or black, the tissues are not receiving enough oxygen. Give CPR.
4. If a broken neck is *not* suspected, turn the victim on his side or stomach; his head should be lower than his feet. This will ensure that vomitus will not obstruct his airway. *It is of paramount importance to maintain an open, unobstructed airway*. Remove any false or broken teeth, mucus, blood, or vomit from the mouth.
5. If a broken neck *is* suspected, the patient must *not* be moved without adequate splinting of the

neck (see diagram). Do *not* bend or twist the neck. Lift the lower jaw forward in order to prevent airway obstruction by the tongue, which will tend to drop backward.

6. Do *not* administer pain medications to an unconscious victim.
7. Do *not* give food or liquids orally to an unconscious victim.
8. Monitor the blood pressure, pulse, respirations per minute, fluid intake by intravenous (IV) route, and urinary output. See "Procedures" chapter for various how-to's.
9. Unconsciousness that lasts over 24 hours is obviously a grave prognostic sign. To keep the victim's vital functions operating properly will require consummate skill and attention to details, foremost being airway maintenance. You cannot realistically expect to perform more than the above measures while aboard a boat at sea.
10. Remember—*record everything.*

7.2 Convulsions (Seizures)

Convulsions may result in a loss of consciousness due to epilepsy, head injury, hemorrhage, tumor, or sustained high fever. It is difficult to predict the occurrence or reoccurrence of seizures, but the following guidelines will be helpful:

TREATMENT:

1. Insert a padded tongue blade between the patient's teeth to prevent bites to the tongue. Do *not* put your fingers into someone's mouth while a seizure is taking place.
2. Protect the patient from hitting his/her head on hard objects.

3. Administer medication to control seizure activity: Valium, 10 mg IM, or Dilantin, 300 mg IM.
4. The patient will usually be sleepy when seizure activity subsides, so allow for uninterrupted rest or sleep.

7.3 Head Injury

Any injury to the head may produce injury to the brain, with or without skull fracture. Whether someone is "knocked out" does not determine the severity of the injury; brain injury may have occurred even when the blow to the head seemed minor, and regardless of the presence or absence of swelling of the scalp. Unless an obvious deformity in the shape of the head exists, and since there will be no X-ray facilities, other signs must be used to help diagnose a skull fracture.

Since the brain can be damaged in varying degrees of severity, it is helpful to define some terms. A concussion occurs from a blow to the skull, and may cause a temporary loss of consciousness and memory and a confused state, but no permanent brain damage occurs. More serious bruising of the brain occurs when blood vessels of the brain are injured. Since there is little room for an accumulation of blood under the skull, any clots that form cause pressure on the brain tissue.

SIGNS AND SYMPTOMS:

Any or all of the following may be present:

1. Drainage from the ears or nose of a clear, water-like fluid, or blood drainage
2. Black eyes
3. Pupils of the eyes not equal in size. Uneven pupil size, with one pupil that does not react when a flashlight is shined equally in the eyes.

4. The eyes may not focus normally. They should not "wander," and both should point in the same direction as the patient looks around.
5. Weakness or paralysis, if the limbs are unequal in strength, or one side of the face sags, or the patient stumbles or staggers or is generally not coordinated
6. Patient may not waken normally after sleeping, or he/she won't awaken at all (coma), or wakes but is unusually drowsy, stuporous, or mentally confused, cannot talk, or can talk but slurs speech. (A child will often be sleepy after a head injury, but can easily be roused.)
7. Any of the following may also indicate severe brain damage:
   a. Increased drowsiness
   b. Persistent or increasingly severe headache
   c. Persistent vomiting
   d. Slowing of the pulse
   e. Convulsions (seizures)
   f. A change from the usual personality or behavior pattern
   g. Marked restlessness, overactivity, or combativeness
   h. Loss of coordination; uses common objects inappropriately

Note: Sometimes, one or more of the above will occur, then go away. Sometimes, symptoms do not show up for as long as two to three months, but that is uncommon.

TREATMENT:
1. *Airway maintenance.* Remove any false teeth, vomitus, or mucus from the airway, and position the head lower than the body, so that if vomiting

occurs, spontaneous drainage will be out of the mouth and not down into the lungs.
2. Administer CPR if necessary; see section 2.1.
3. Control any bleeding; cover any open wounds.
4. Keep the victim's neck straight and lash him/her to a board so that their body is moved as a single unit; this will prevent further damage in the event there is also a neck injury.

Note: These victims should be transferred to a medical facility as quickly as possible.

7.4 Hyperventilation

As a cause of unconsciousness, hyperventilation is most often caused by emotional upset, which results in fainting.

SIGNS AND SYMPTOMS:
1. Rapid breathing, shortness of breath, and increased pulse
2. "Tingling" and spasms of the fingers and toes
3. Anxiety
4. Dizziness or light-headedness
5. A numbness around the mouth may be present.

TREATMENT:
1. Instruct the patient to breathe *slowly* into a paper (not plastic) bag held over the face. This increases the carbon dioxide level in the blood, which will help alleviate signs and symptoms. Continue this for 5–10 minutes.
2. Reassurance and rest are important supportive measures.

7.5 Diabetes

Any discussion of diabetes in this limited context must assume that the ship's company will have prior knowledge of someone's diabetic condition.

7.5a Diabetic Coma

SIGNS AND SYMPTOMS:

1. Confusion
2. Dry, flushed skin
3. Dry tongue
4. Labored breathing

TREATMENT:

This is a very grave condition, and its treatment requires medical attention beyond the scope of this text. *Seek medical assistance immediately.*

7.5b Hypoglycemia—Insulin Reaction

Hypoglycemia, or low blood sugar, is a common medical condition. Any known diabetic who displays the following symptoms, whether he takes insulin or an oral antidiabetic agent, may be having a hypoglycemic reaction.

SIGNS AND SYMPTOMS:

1. Nervousness
2. Rapid pulse
3. Sweating
4. Shallow breathing
5. Confusion
6. At times, unconsciousness

TREATMENT:

1. Administer sugar, either by giving a candy bar or by putting 1–2 teaspoonsful of sugar in a glass of juice or water.
2. If the patient cannot swallow, an IV (intravenous) infusion of 5% dextrose should be administered. See "Procedures," sections 15.1 and 15.2.

8. Burns

Burns are classified as first-degree, second-degree, or third-degree. They must be evaluated by this classification and by the amount of body surface involved.

—First-degree: Produces redness of the skin
—Second-degree: Produces redness of the skin and some blisters
—Third-degree: A full thickness of the skin is burned and may appear pale, white, brown, or black. There is a loss of pain sensation to pinprick in the area.

If the patient has either moderate or severe burns, seek further medical treatment immediately. To evaluate these burns use the following guidelines:

Severe burns:

1. Third-degree burns of face, hands, and feet
2. Third-degree burns of 10% of the body surface
3. Second-degree burns of 30% of the body surface

Moderate burns:

1. Third-degree burns of 2–10% of the body surface, and not involving face, hands, and feet
2. Second-degree burns of 15–30% of the body surface, and not involving face, hands, or feet
3. First-degree burns of 50–75% of body surface, and not involving face, hands, and feet

Minor burns:

1. Third-degree burns of less than 2% of the body surface
2. Second-degree burns of less than 15% of the body surface
3. First-degree burns of less than 20% of the body surface, not including face, hands, and feet

The "Rule of Nines" is the general guide used to evaluate the percentage of body area burned. "Nines" means 9% of the body surface. Burns should be evaluated by this rule. See diagram.

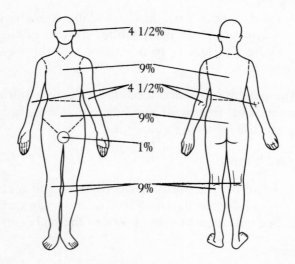

The rule of nines. Calculate the amount of body surface burned as a percentage.

IMMEDIATE TREATMENT FOR ALL BURNS:

1. Make sure adequate breathing is taking place. Burns of the face or neck may result in respi-

---

ratory distress. If breathing is not adequate, administer CPR.

2. Apply cold, wet compresses for 5–10 minutes. Further application of compresses may produce shivering, which is not desirable.
3. Administer pain medication if needed: Demerol, 50 mg IM may be given, or one Tylenol #3 orally.
4. Flush (irrigate) the burn area with fresh water. Continue for 20–30 minutes. This is especially true of any chemical burn of the eyes. *Do not* use butter, Vaseline, or other compresses. Forget vinegar or baking soda applications; *pour water, water, and more water over the area.* Seawater is acceptable if fresh water is unavailable or in short supply.
5. Cover the burn area with Silvadene cream or Furacin ointment. These are antimicrobials.
6. Apply a sterile dressing.
7. Keep the area clean and dry. The dressing may be changed daily, when new antimicrobial cream is again lightly applied.
8. Do not open the fluid-filled blisters associated with second-degree burns.

9. Swimming and Diving Emergencies

9.1 Near Drowning

Drowning is a common cause of accidental death. Lack of oxygen leads to loss of consciousness, cardiac arrest, and brain damage. Hypothermia may also complicate the situation, and may actually be the precipitating cause of drowning.

IMMEDIATE TREATMENT:

1. Begin CPR; see section 2.1.
2. Do not attempt to drain water from the patient first. Circulation and ventilation are the priorities.

Although treatment of the drowning victim is currently controversial, I would suggest the following guidelines for the treatment of a saltwater drowning victim:

1. Follow the two steps listed above under "Immediate Treatment."
2. If available, administer Lasix, 80 mg IM, if the breathing is noisy or "gurgly." Do *not* give Lasix to a freshwater drowning victim.
3. Administer an antibiotic, such as penicillin, 600,000 units IM, or ampicillin, 500 mg IM.
4. Turn the victim onto his stomach when spontaneous breathing has resumed.

5. Keep the patient warm.
6. Do not give the patient solid food; small sips of water or hot tea may be given.

9.2 Air Embolism (Decompression Sickness; "The Bends")

Air embolism is a common hazard in scuba diving, and can be deadly. Air bubbles form in blood vessels and act as plugs to prevent oxygen from reaching body tissues, sometimes causing heart or brain damage.

SIGNS AND SYMPTOMS:

1. Pain or aching in muscles, especially the shoulder, as well as in joints or tendons
2. Froth in the mouth and nose
3. Blotching or itching of the skin, or a tingling feeling or numbness
4. Chest pain and difficulty breathing
5. Nausea and vomiting, along with abdominal pain
6. Dizziness
7. Difficulty seeing; blurred vision
8. Headache
9. Paralysis or coma

TREATMENT:

1. Administer oxygen, if available.
2. Find a recompression chamber. If no recompression chamber is available, the patient should be returned to recompression depth—*only if able to do so*—and kept there for the length of time indicated by the timetable for decompression diving.

After the above steps have been successful:

1. Administer oral or intravenous (IV) fluids. (If IV,
   see sections 15.1 and 15.2. Use lactated Ringer's
   solution or 5% dextrose solution.) This will aid
   rehydration in the victim.
2. Administer two aspirin, twice a day.
3. Administer a steroid, such as hydrocortisone, 100
   mg IM.

Note: To prevent air embolism, use the decompression
tables in the U.S. Navy Diving Manual. However, it should
be noted that this manual is not infallible. *Slow ascent* from
any dive is necessary. If a diving accident occurs while
inside the U.S., a physician may be contacted at any time
by calling the Divers Alert Network, telephone (919) 684-
8111, (919) 684-5514, or (919) 684-2948.

9.3 Contact with the Marine Environment

9.3a Portuguese Man-of-War; Jellyfish; Fire Coral
SIGNS AND SYMPTOMS:

1. Linear, spiral lesions from the tentacles,
   purplish-red in color
2. Severe pain
3. Itching, either localized or generalized
4. Respiratory distress if contact is severe

TREATMENT:

1. Administer CPR if necessary; see section 2.1.
2. Neutralize the toxin with vinegar or the commercial product Stingose. Vinegar will neutralize
   the discharge of the nematocyst—the stinging
   cell at the end of a tentacle. The following, although commonly used by many people, stimulate nematocyst discharge, *and should be avoided:*

meat tenderizer, ammonia, alcohol (either rubbing or liquor), or baking soda.
3. Administer Benadryl (an antihistamine), 50 mg, either IM or orally.
4. Administer pain medication; either Demerol, 50 mg IM, or Tylenol #3 orally.
5. Administer Decadron, 4 mg orally. Decadron is a steroid medication sometimes used to counteract allergic reactions.
6. Apply hot towels to the area.

9.3b Sea Urchins

TREATMENT:
1. Embedded spines are often difficult to remove. Soak the area in vinegar 4 times a day to help dissolve them.
2. If infection occurs, take an antibiotic orally: penicillin or ampicillin, 250 mg 4 times a day.

9.3c Poisonous Fish Spines

For a commercial fisherman or cannery worker, being punctured by a fish spine is an almost daily occurrence. However, the pleasure-boater or weekend fisherman is not immune to fish-spine accidents, or their sometimes toxic effects.

TREATMENT:
1. I have asked many people what they do to treat fish-spine injuries, and received just as many answers. However, the common denominator in the immediate treatment is to soak the affected area in hot water with chlorine bleach, with PhisoHex, or betadine added, for 1–2 hours.
2. Apply a topical antibiotic, such as Polymyxin, to the area 4 times a day.

3. If a boil or red streaks indicating a localized infection appear, or if continued swelling or pain persist, begin a broad-spectrum antibiotic, such as penicillin or ampicillin, 250 mg 4 times a day.

9.3d Stingray Wounds

SIGNS AND SYMPTOMS:

1. Severe pain or stinging in wounded area
2. Possible systemic symptoms of nausea, vomiting or diarrhea, rapid pulse, sweating; rarely, shock and death
3. The wound is swollen and red, with a laceration or puncture.

TREATMENT:

1. Prompt and copious cleaning of the area to wash out the venom from the spine of the stingray, which is left in the tissue whether the spine is embedded or not.
2. Antibiotic treatment, although controversial, will probably help. Use penicillin, ampicillin, or Keflex, 250 mg 4 times a day.
3. Pain medication may be needed, such as Demerol, 50 mg IM, or one Tylenol #3, orally.
4. Keep the affected area elevated.

10. Contact with Poisonous Insects, Animals, and Snakes

10.1 Bee, Wasp, and Hornet Stings

SIGNS AND SYMPTOMS:

1. A small, red area with swelling, itching, and heat
2. In a *severe reaction*, the above, plus sneezing, difficulty breathing, difficulty swallowing, generalized weakness, nausea, vomiting or diarrhea, and generalized itching over the entire body
3. Death may occur in one of four ways in a very severe reaction:
   a. Many stings, up to 400
   b. Localization of the many stings
   c. IV (intravenous) stings
   d. Hypersensitivity reaction; anaphylactic shock due to a severe allergic reaction is probably the most common cause of death.

TREATMENT:

1. Gently remove stinger, if present.
2. Apply ice to the area.
3. Elevate the involved limb.

TREATMENT OF SEVERE REACTION:

1. All of the above, plus CPR if necessary
2. Administer adrenalin (epinephrine), 1:1000 so-

73

lution, in an adult dose of 0.3–0.5 cc, subcutaneously (SQ). See "Procedures," section 15.4.
3. Administer Benadryl (an antihistamine), 50 mg IM or orally.
4. Administer Decadron (a steroid medication), 4 mg IM or orally.
5. Administer antibiotics, such as penicillin or ampicillin, 250 mg 4 times a day.
6. There are bee-sting kits available commercially. One should be kept aboard if a crew member is known to have a hypersensitivity to bees, wasps, hornets, etc. These kits are either the Ana-Kit or Nelco-kit, the dose of the 1:1000 solution being adrenalin, 0.5 cc subcutaneously (SQ) for 2 doses.

10.2 Ants, Flies, Chiggers, Mosquitoes

SIGNS AND SYMPTOMS:

1. Redness
2. Swelling or welts
3. Itching

TREATMENT:

1. Apply baking-soda paste or Calamine lotion to neutralize the toxin.
2. If the above are unavailable, apply cool compresses.
3. Scrub the area with soap and water.
4. If infection occurs, begin oral antibiotics such as penicillin or ampicillin, 250 mg 4 times a day.
5. A topical steroid spray or cream, such as Decaspray or hydrocortisone cream, applied to the affected area 4 times a day may be helpful.

10.3 Ticks

TREATMENT:

1. *Do not* try to pull the tick out. See below.
2. Cover the tick with Vaseline; this will smother it, and it should let go. If Vaseline is unavailable, use gasoline, kerosene, or oil to smother the tick.
3. If the tick does not let go, then gently pry it out with tweezers.
4. Wash the area thoroughly with PhisoHex or betadine.
5. If infection, headache, malaise, fever chills, skin rash, muscle aches, or abdominal pain occur, begin antibiotics, preferably tetracycline, 250 mg 4 times a day for 10 days.

PREVENTION:

1. Check daily for ticks if you're in an area known to harbor them.
2. Wear clothing that covers the body, such as long-sleeved shirts, long pants, hats, socks, etc.

10.4 Snakebites

There are two general categories of poisonous snakes in North America:

1. Pit viper (rattlesnake, cottonmouth, copperhead, water moccasin): Characterized by a pit between the eye and the nostril, one or more sets of fangs, vertical pupils, a triangular head, a single anal subcaudal plate, and there may or may not be rattles
2. Coral snakes: These are usually red and yellow with a black nose. The following mnemonic is

helpful to remember in attempting to identify a coral snake:

Red on Yellow—Kill the Fellow
Red on Black—Venom Lack

There are over 2000 types of snake in the world—400 are poisonous. An attempt should be made to identify the snake.

SIGNS AND SYMPTOMS OF SNAKEBITE:
1. Pain and swelling at the site
2. One or two fang marks
3. If severe: nausea, vomiting, slurred speech, variable heart rate, or shock.
4. Tiny hemorrhages into the skin at the site

TREATMENT:
There is much controversy, and many opinionated articles have been written about snakebite treatment. The following represents, I feel, the most commonly accepted suggestion for treatment:

1. Apply tourniquets above and below the site, but *do not* restrict circulation.
2. After cleaning the skin with an antiseptic, such as PhisoHex or betadine solution, cut X-marked incisions over the fang marks and suck the venom out with a bulb syringe, if one is available, or by mouth if necessary. The latter method is less favorable because of the possibility of introducing infection. The incisions should be ⅛ to ¼ inch in depth and about ½ inch in length, and placed over each fang mark.
3. Administer antivenin (if available) when identification of a poisonous snake is positive, *and*

the patient is *not* allergic to horse serum. Follow instructions and procedures in the snakebite kit.

4. Do not allow the victim to move around. Restrict the movements of other people to reduce anxiety and stress in the patient.
5. Do not give any alcoholic beverages.
6. Do *not* apply ice or cold compresses.
7. Antibiotics for wound infection may be necessary: penicillin or Keflex, 250 mg 4 times a day.

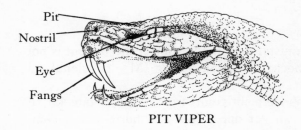

Pit
Nostril
Eye
Fangs

PIT VIPER

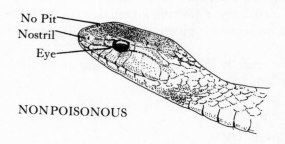

No Pit
Nostril
Eye

NONPOISONOUS

Poisonous snakes have a pit between the eye and nostril, fangs, vertical pupils, and a triangular head.

8. Administer pain medications if necessary: Demerol, 50 mg IM for severe pain, or Tylenol #3 for less severe pain. Do not give aspirin for pain, as aspirin affects the blood's clotting mechanisms (as does the venom from the poisonous snake).

10.5 Spiders

10.5a Black Widow

SIGNS AND SYMPTOMS:

1. Dull pain at the site of the bite
2. Two puncture wounds at site, surrounded by redness and swelling
3. If bite is severe, or if a severe reaction occurs, shock may ensue.

TREATMENT:

1. Apply icepack to the site.
2. Administer pain medication if the patient is not in shock: Demerol, 50 mg IM, or Tylenol #3 orally.
3. Administer antivenin from a spider-bite kit, if you can get one. This is a horse-serum compound, and a severe allergic reaction may occur. Test for allergy, following instructions in the kit. If the antivenin is given, one ampule is usually enough.
4. Do *not* treat by incision and drainage; do *not* use a tourniquet.

10.5b Brown Recluse

SIGNS AND SYMPTOMS:

1. Stinging and pain at the site
2. Formation of a blister at the site
3. A rash may occur.
4. A depressed, ulcerated area forms within a week, and subsides within three weeks' time.
5. In severe reactions, fever, chills, malaise, weakness, nausea and vomiting, or joint pain may occur.

78

TREATMENT:

1. Administer Benadryl (an antihistamine), 50 mg IM or orally.
2. Administer pain medication if necessary: Demerol, 50 mg IM, or Tylenol #3 orally.
3. Administer a steroid medication, such as Decadron, 4 mg orally or IM.
4. Administer an antibiotic, such as penicillin, ampicillin, or Keflex, 250 mg 4 times a day.
5. Apply warm compresses to the area.

10.6 Scorpions

SIGNS AND SYMPTOMS:

1. "Pins and needles" sensation
2. No swelling or discoloration
3. If bite is severe: itching of the nose, mouth, and throat; spasms, nausea, and vomiting; seizures (convulsions)
4. Pain in the affected area, which is very sensitive even to light touch

TREATMENT:

1. Apply ice to site.
2. Adminster pain medication if needed: Demerol, 50 mg IM., or Tylenol #3 orally.
3. Administer antivenin if available. This antivenin is *not* a horse-serum extract, so no allergic reaction is expected.
4. Administer Benadryl (an antihistamine), 50 mg IM or orally.

11. Poisoning

Adults and children aboard ship are exposed to the same threats of poisoning—by ingestion, inhalation, injection, or absorption—that exist elsewhere. The *basic principles of management* are to:

1. Maintain the victim's airway if unconsciousness or shock is present.
2. Administer CPR if necessary; see section 2.1.
3. Remove or deactivate the poison before systemic absorption can occur.

In some situations, a clue as to what has happened can be found by observation: Is there an empty pill bottle or fuel container nearby? Is there any unusual smell to the victim or his/her clothing?

Specific categories of poisoning and examples follow:

11.1 Inhaled Poisons

Example: Chemicals, such as carbon tetrachloride, or toxic fumes such as carbon monoxide (watch those heaters down below when the vessel is battened down with little or no ventilation).

SIGNS AND SYMPTOMS OF CARBON MONOXIDE POISONING:

1. Strange or confused behavior
2. Headache
3. Skin color is not a very accurate measure of acute poisoning.

80

TREATMENT:
1. CPR if necessary; see section 2.1
2. Get the victim into fresh air as quickly as possible. Administering oxygen would be helpful, but few vessels have oxygen tanks aboard.

11.2 Absorbed Poisons

This can result from skin or eye contamination from splashed battery acid, or from other acids or alkalis.

TREATMENT:

Copious irrigation with water for at least half an hour, even after any contaminated clothing has been removed.

11.3 Ingested Poisons (not including food poisoning, found in section 11.5)

In any ingestion of a poisonous substance, it is important to determine whether the poison is corrosive or noncorrosive, as the treatments for each differ. Corrosive (caustic) substances, such as acids, alkalis, ammonia, or petroleum distillates (paint thinner, lighter fluid, gasoline, etc.) cause the following:

SIGNS AND SYMPTOMS:
1. Painful burning of the lips, mouth, and esophagus may occur.
2. Difficulty breathing
3. Possible drooling at the mouth

TREATMENT:
1. *Do not induce vomiting.*
2. Give 1–2 glasses of milk to dilute the poison.

3. When a petroleum distillate of some kind has been ingested, a chemical pneumonia can occur. The signs of this are fever, cough, difficulty breathing, and other signs of pneumonia as covered in section 4.3c. Although the treatment is controversial, I would suggest giving the patient an antibiotic, such as penicillin, ampicillin, or Keflex, in a dose of 250–500 mg every 6 hours.

If a *noncorrosive* substance has been ingested, attempt to induce vomiting by giving syrup of Ipecac, 30 cc orally, followed by 4–5 glasses of water; or by sticking the index finger down the throat. *Remember: Do not induce vomiting in an unconscious person or in someone having a seizure.*

11.4 Injected Poisons

Examples of this are stings by bees, wasps, etc. See sections 10.1, 10.5, and 10.6.

11.5 Food Poisoning

Although food poisoning really comes under the heading of "Ingested Poisons," section 11.3 above, we'll consider various causes of food poisoning separately, in the following categories:

a. Bacterial poisoning
b. Fish poisoning, including ciguatera and scombroid
c. Shellfish poisoning

11.5a Bacterial Food Poisoning

SIGNS AND SYMPTOMS:

1. Nausea and vomiting
2. Diarrhea

3. General weakness
4. Abdominal pain
5. Fever

TREATMENT:

1. Administer pain medication if cramps are severe: Demerol, 50–75 mg IM.
2. If ingestion was recent and vomiting has not occurred, syrup of Ipecac may be given; dosage is 30 cc orally, followed by 4–5 glasses of water. Usually, however, nausea and/or vomiting will be taking place, so syrup of Ipecac won't be needed.
3. Oral fluids should be given only if tolerated, and in small quantities. Intravenous (IV) fluids may be required.
4. Since the symptoms and treatments are similar to those covered in Chapter 5, "Abdominal Pain," refer to sections 5.1, 5.2, and 5.4 for more specific treatments.

11.5b Fish Poisoning (Scombroid)

The fish involved here are tuna, mackerel, bonito, albacore, skipjack, and dolphin fish. The main cause of poisoning is inadequate fish preservation. When these fish spoil, the high histadine level in their flesh and muscles is acted upon by bacteria, which change the histadine into a histaminelike substance called saurine, which then causes the following:

SYMPTOMS (can occur within minutes of eating the fish):

1. Redness of the face and upper torso (like a sunburn)
2. Severe headache
3. Red eyes

4. Dry mouth
5. Nausea, or vomiting, or diarrhea
6. Abdominal pain
7. Welts on the skin and intense itching
8. Palpitations

TREATMENT:

1. Tagamet, 300 mg IV over several minutes, will cause the symptoms to abate. If IV Tagamet is unavailable, then one 300 mg Tagamet tablet can be given orally. If Tagamet is unavailable, then:
2. Benadryl, 50 mg IM or orally, acts as an antihistamine.

PREVENTION:

Eat fish promptly, or preserve properly by canning or freezing. Cooking does *not* destroy the toxin. *Remember:* Any fish that looks or smells bad *is* bad.

Fish Poisoning (Ciguatera)

Almost any fish can produce symptoms of ciguatera poisoning, and edibility cannot be predicted according to whether you have eaten a particular kind of fish before without ill effects. Fish such as jack, herring, grouper, seabass, wrasse, snapper, parrotfish, and barracuda may eat smaller fish that have eaten the dinoflagellate (a poisonous microscopic marine animal) that produces the ciguatera.

SYMPTOMS:

1. Tingling or numbness of the lips, tongue, hands, or feet
2. Dizziness
3. Nausea or vomiting, with abdominal cramps
4. Muscle and joint aches and pains

5. Headache
6. Blurred vision
7. Skin disorders similar to allergic food reaction (itching, skin wheals, redness)
8. In very severe cases, muscle weakness, paralysis, seizures, or death may occur.

DIAGNOSIS:

No reliable test is available; base your diagnosis on a history of recent fish ingestion and some or all of the above symptoms.

TREATMENT:

1. CPR if necessary; see section 2.1
2. Empty the stomach by giving syrup of Ipecac, 30 cc orally, followed by 4–5 glasses of water, or force vomiting (finger down throat).
3. Give fluids and vitamin supplements in less serious reactions to encourage body healing and possibly lessen the chance of later neurologic disorder.
4. During the acute phase, pain medication may be required: Demerol, 50–75 mg IM.

PREVENTION:

Eat smaller fish, not larger ones. Avoid the roe, liver, and intestines. *Remember:* No method of cooking fish destroys the toxin; nor does drying, freezing, or pickling.

11.5c Shellfish Poisoning

Shellfish poisoning can occur in conjunction with a "red tide," when seawater appears red because of the large amount of dinoflagellates in the area. The molluscs (various kinds of mussels and clams) we eat store the poison, which then acts as a toxin in our system.

SIGNS AND SYMPTOMS:

1. Nausea, vomiting, or diarrhea, associated with abdominal pain
2. An allergic reaction manifested by hives, headaches, increase in the pulse rate, or difficulty breathing
3. Tingling of the lips and face, and numbness in those areas may occur
4. Difficulty swallowing
5. Joint aches and pains
6. Generalized weakness, and, in some cases, paralysis

TREATMENT:

1. CPR if necessary; see section 2.1
2. No specific antidote exists.
3. Empty the stomach by giving syrup of Ipecac, 30 cc orally, followed by 4–5 glasses of water, or force vomiting (finger down throat).

Remember: Poisonous shellfish cannot be recognized by odor, color, or general appearance. Tide level makes no difference as to the suitability of shellfish for harvesting and eating.

12. The Offshore Environment

12.1 Heat Exhaustion/Prostration

Maintenance of our constant body temperature is governed by heat gain and heat loss.

Heat gain:

1. Radiation: Sun
2. Convection: Air current; wind velocity
3. Conduction: Direct contact (as in a hot bath)
4. Internal: Our cellular metabolism and muscle activity (as in exercise and shivering). This accounts for about 2000–5000 calories per day.

Heat loss:

1. Radiation: An increase in energy output transmits heat to the environment.
2. Convection: Occurs when air temperature is lower than body temperature. Wind increases this.
3. Conduction: direct contact with cold water or ice
4. Evaporation: This is the main way we lose heat, especially by sweating. We can lose 1.5 liters per hour if we are unacclimatized, up to 3 liters per hour acclimatized, and it may take the body a week to adjust to a new environment.

SIGNS AND SYMPTOMS:

1. Generalized weakness; may feel faint or collapse
2. Enlarged pupils

3. Headache
4. Loss of appetite; may have nausea or vomiting
5. Fast and weak pulse
6. Skin is pale and feels clammy and cold (A red flush to the skin may indicate heatstroke.)
7. Shallow breathing
8. Muscle cramps, especially of the legs; may be quite severe
9. Mental status changes: impaired judgment, fatigue, and anxiety
10. Temperature may be within normal limits, not greatly elevated

TREATMENT:

1. Move the person to a cooler area and remove or loosen clothing.
2. The person should lie on his/her back with the legs slightly raised.
3. Administer fluids and salt tablets (5 grams of salt is our usual daily maintenance).
4. Apply cool compresses to the forehead.
5. Fan the person. Evaporation is the most effective way to lose heat.

Remember: Check your urine output and color. If you're urinating regularly and your urine is clear, your hydration is OK. If your urine output is down, and your urine is dark yellow, drink more fluids.

12.2 Heatstroke (Sunstroke)

A high temperature is *not* needed for excessive heat accumulation to occur. If exercise is vigorous enough, heatstroke can occur at relatively low air temperatures, especially if the humidity is high. Most people cannot rid the body of more than 600 calories per hour, and an increase in exercise will then lead to an increase in heat retention.

In this context, we'll consider heatstroke as a derangement of brain function secondary to an elevated temperature. Whether the patient is comatose, delirious, or just confused depends on the circumstances involved and the individual patient.

PREDISPOSING FACTORS:

1. Infection (such as pneumonia)
2. Skin diseases
3. Alcoholism, especially when the person is severely agitated
4. Impaired cardiovascular function, often in elderly people (the heart and skin both help to promote heat loss)
5. Dehydration
6. Potassium depletion
7. Obesity
8. Inappropriate choice of clothing
9. Medications or drugs (e.g., thyroid, PCP, amphetamines, LSD, phenothiazines, antihistamines, diabetes medicines)
10. Diabetes
11. High ambient temperature
12. High humidity
13. Little or no wind velocity
14. Overexertion

SIGNS AND SYMPTOMS:

During vigorous exercise in the wrong situation, many people will have no warning of heatstroke. Although early signs like malaise, weakness, loss of appetite, or disorientation may appear, also look for:

1. High temperature
2. Red flush to the skin, which is very hot and dry
3. Strong, throbbing, and rapid pulse (over 110 beats per minute)
4. Headache and/or confusion
5. Dizziness; may feel faint or collapse
6. Rapid breathing
7. Abdominal discomfort; nausea and/or vomiting
8. Dry mouth

TREATMENT:

1. Wrap the patient in cold, wet sheets.
2. Fan the patient; this is the most effective method of evaporation.
3. Sponge the skin with cool water.
4. Stop cooling measures when the temperature comes down to the 101–102-degree range. Record temperatures every 30 minutes during that time.
5. Administer oral fluids if the patient is conscious, and give salt tablets. Give 3–4 glasses of water with ½ teaspoon of salt every 15 minutes for 45 minutes (3 times).
6. Aspirin or Tylenol is of no benefit, and should not be given.
7. If the body temperature continues to go up because of shivering, or if the person has a seizure (convulsion) or is not rational, administer an IM injection of either Valium, 10 mg, or Thorazine, 50 mg.

PREVENTION:

1. Protection from the sun is of utmost importance. Light clothing and a hat should be worn.
2. Our daily maintenance dose of salt is 5 grams.

Usually, the salt in our food is adequate, but in especially hot conditions, enteric-coated salt tablets may be taken.
3. Encourage fluid intake, especially throughout daylight hours. Drink at least 4 quarts of liquid a day when sweating is constant.
4. Avoid alcoholic and caffeinated beverages when you are increasing your fluid intake on hot, sunny days. Water and fruit juices are better.
5. Cool showers with seawater will help.
6. Remember to keep track of your hydration status by paying attention to your urine output and color.

12.3 Cold Exposure (Hypothermia)

Cold temperatures, cold water, and brisk wind pose a definite threat to the unprepared crew member. Properly insulated clothing, including long underwear and insulated jackets, socks, gloves, wool hats with ear protection, or even "survival suits" for anticipated cold, heavy-weather sailing should be mandatory for well-prepared mariners.

SIGNS AND SYMPTOMS:

An overlap of symptoms occurs, but progressive muscular, brain, and circulatory impairment occurs as follows:

1. Muscular reactions such as uncontrollable shivering, short episodes of violent shivering, goose bumps all over the body, rigid muscles, fumbling hands, or an unsteady walk
2. Vague, slow, slurred, or incoherent speech
3. Lapses of memory, reduced judgment, reduced ability to reason
4. Irrational behavior

5. Abnormally low body temperature. Since regular thermometers don't record very low temperatures, the evaluation of hypothermia will depend on the above signs and symptoms.
6. Drowsiness, lethargy, apathy, unconsciousness. Some victims of hypothermia may appear to be dead.

TREATMENT:

1. Administer CPR if necessary; see section 2.1.
2. Try to keep the person warm and dry; go below where it is warm immediately, and replace wet articles of clothing.
3. Cover the person with blankets and place hot packs on the chest and abdomen. Do not put hot packs on the arms or legs. Do not give the hypothermia victim up for dead, as resuscitation may be a lengthy process.
4. Do not allow the person to smoke; this causes constriction of the blood vessels.
5. Administer hot cocoa or other hot liquid.
6. Let the person get lots of rest.

PREVENTION:

1. Adequate clothing
2. Awareness of the *early* signs of hypothermia
3. Adequate food, water, and salt intake in a situation where hypothermia may occur. These measures help to hydrate the body and allow adequate body energy to maintain constant body temperature.
4. Reduce unnecessary physical activity.

12.4 Frostbite

To avoid frostbite, cover and/or protect the areas of the body that are most easily exposed to cold, such as ears, nose, fingers, and toes. See "Prevention," under section 12.3 above.

SIGNS AND SYMPTOMS:
1. A "burning" sensation, becoming a feeling of "pins and needles," eventually followed by stiffness and loss of feeling in the affected part
2. An area of skin that is whitish in color and does not change to red or pink after pressure has been applied, and that feels stiff and hard to the touch

TREATMENT:
1. *Do not* rub, chafe, or move the frostbitten extremity.
2. *Do not* apply snow or ice in an attempt to thaw out the affected part in cold water.
3. *Do* administer tepid (warm) water soaks. *Do not* use hot water. Continue warm soaks for 45–60 minutes.
4. Pain medication may be needed, such as Demerol, 50 mg IM.
5. Superficial frostbite generally does not lead to permanent tissue damage, but itching, tingling, and red, sensitive skin may reoccur upon reexposure to cold.
6. Administer warm, nonalcoholic beverages, such as hot cocoa, broth, or herbal tea. Avoid caffeine-containing coffees and teas, as these may stimulate further blood-vessel constriction.
7. Do not allow the victim to smoke; this will also cause blood-vessel constriction.

8. Look for signs of infection in the frostbitten area; if infected, a broad-spectrum antibiotic, such as ampicillin, 250 mg orally, 4 times a day, may be given.
9. Gently apply sterile dressings to the area, and change them daily.

13. Emergency Childbirth; Miscarriage

13.1 Emergency Childbirth

Ideally, an expectant mother will have optimum surroundings and conditions in which to deliver her newborn. However, the normal gestation period is an inexact chronometer. Babies are supposed to be born about 40 weeks after conception, but sometimes these new crew members sign on between the thirty-fifth and fortieth weeks of their mother's pregnancy. If you're in a situation where childbirth is imminent, the following guidelines will assist you:

SUPPLIES USED IN DELIVERY (See section 15.9, "How to Sterilize Equipment"):

1. Sterile towels
2. Sterile clamps to clamp umbilical cord
3. Sterile scissors to cut umbilical cord
4. Warm (boil and let cool) water for cleansing
5. Sterile gloves
6. Sterile pan or bucket to be used in the delivery of the placenta
7. Blankets and aluminum foil to wrap the baby
8. Suction bulb to clear mucus from the baby's nose and mouth

Remember: Mothers have been delivering babies for thousands of years; you just may not have had the chance to help before. *Stay calm!*

LABOR:

Generally, the period of labor for the first baby is longer than for the succeeding ones. Labor pains are characterized by stomachache and backache, and become more frequent and regular as labor progresses.

1. Find a comfortable place for the mother.
2. Use a clean sheet under her (with a foul-weather jacket under the sheet) and have good lighting available.
3. Wash your hands well; also wash the mother's pubic hair and birth canal area.
4. Encourage relaxation and have the mother take long, deep breaths through her mouth, inhaling and exhaling rhythmically.
5. If a bowel movement is passed, gently wipe away from the birth canal area and wash with soap and water.

DELIVERY:

1. As the baby's head begins to push out of the vagina with each contraction, gently push against it so that it will not forcefully "explode" from the vagina. The mother should not push when the pain occurs; gradual stretching of the birth canal and slow birth of the baby's head is desired.
2. After the head appears, check to see if the umbilical cord is wrapped around the baby's neck. If so, attempt to slip the cord gently over the baby's head. If this cannot be done because the cord is wrapped too tightly, clamp the cord in

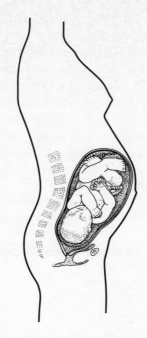

Position of full-term fetus

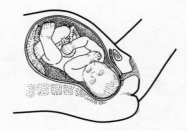

First stage of labor

two places and cut the cord between the clamps. Then unwrap the cord from around the neck.

3. Remember to support the head at all times. The baby will be slippery, so be careful.

4. After the head is clear of the birth canal, the baby will usually rotate to the right or left, and the upper shoulder then usually follows. At this point, delivery of the rest of the infant should occur without problem.

5. Keep the baby's head lower than its body, and gently suction the mucus and blood from its nose and mouth.

6. As the umbilical cord is still attached, clamp it

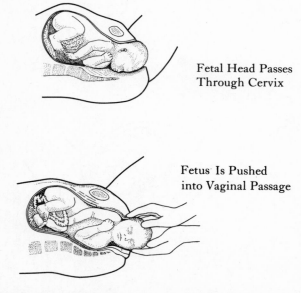

Fetal Head Passes
Through Cervix

Fetus Is Pushed
into Vaginal Passage

Prevent forceful expulsion of baby's head by gently supporting it. As the head appears, check to see whether the umbilical cord is wrapped around the baby's neck. After the head is delivered, the upper shoulder usually follows. The rest of the infant then rapidly emerges.

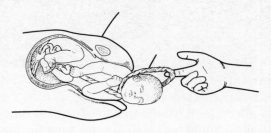

Position of the umbilical cord wrapped around the baby's neck. Gently lift and unwrap the cord.

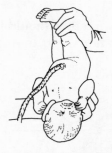

Hold the baby's head lower than its body. The umbilical cord may then be clamped.

in two places several inches from the baby's navel and then cut the cord between the clamps.

7. Wrap the baby in blankets and then cover him/her in aluminum foil in order to retain body heat.

AFTERBIRTH:

1. After about 15–30 minutes the placenta (afterbirth) usually separates from the uterus, and can be removed from the vaginal area.
2. Don't pull on the cord in order to rush delivery of the placenta.
3. Don't be frightened if bleeding at the birth canal occurs.

4. The lower part of the mother's abdomen can be gently massaged. This will help the uterus to firm up.
5. Following passage of the placenta, give the mother an injection of Methergine, 0.2 mg IM (one ampule). This helps constrict the smooth muscles of the uterus and thereby stops uterine bleeding.
6. Any small tears at the entrance to the vagina can be treated simply by cleansing the area, dressing with sterile bandages, and then leaving them alone.
7. After resting, the mother should be encouraged to sit up in her bunk and move around when able.

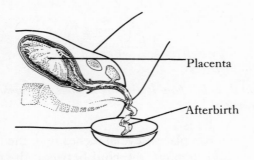

The placental membrane eventually separates from the uterus and may be accompanied by a gush of blood.

CARE OF THE NEW BABY:

1. *Keep warm.* After the cord has been tied, wrap the baby in clean, dry clothes and then wrap aluminum foil or blankets around him/her to help prevent heat loss.
2. Keep the baby on its belly, with the head slightly lower than the rest of its body.

3. Allow the baby to rest.
4. Change soiled and wet clothing every 3–4 hours or when necessary.
5. In general, keep the baby as quiet and undisturbed as possible.

FEEDING THE BABY:

1. Newborn infants may be put to the breast soon after delivery to receive the mother's highly nutritious colostrum. Nursing at this time will also improve uterine contractions.
2. The infant may be nursed every 3–4 hours, or on demand.
3. The mother's full milk flow may not be established for 2–3 days after delivery.
4. As a supplement, baby's milk formula (powder, concentrate, or full-strength) may be given. Follow the directions on the package closely.
5. Occasional suplemental feedings of sugar water may be given. Add 1 tsp of sugar to 8 oz boiled water; allow to cool.

Note: Complications of delivery for both baby and mother are outside the scope of this text.

13.2 Miscarriage

Vaginal bleeding in early pregnancy is not uncommon. Bed rest is usually all that is needed, as bleeding will usually stop spontaneously. Signs that miscarriage (spontaneous abortion) may occur are as follows:

1. Bleeding that does not stop spontaneously with bed rest.
2. Lower abdominal pains and cramps.

TREATMENT:

1. Encourage bed rest.
2. Encourage increased fluid intake.

IF MISCARRIAGE DOES OCCUR:

A sudden worsening of vaginal bleeding may indicate that spontaneous abortion has occurred.

1. Administer pain medication: Demerol, 50 mg IM.
2. Administer Methergine, one tablet orally ($^1/_{320}$ grain) to encourage contractions in order to expel the dead fetus and placenta.

14. Trauma

14.1 Back or Neck Injury

If numbness of the extremities, weakness, or paralysis is present, or develops later, as a result of a back or neck injury, medical assistance must be obtained as soon as possible. A backboard should be used to immobilize the victim, and precautions taken to immobilize the neck so that it doesn't rotate to the side.

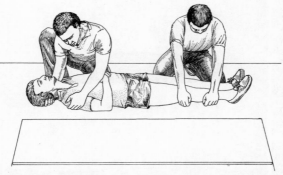

Care must be taken to keep the head, neck, and body in straight alignment, thereby preventing the neck from flexing. Note the support under the victim's head before rolling him.

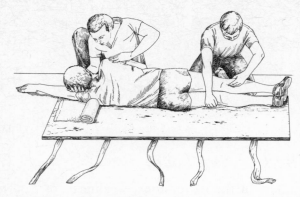

Gently roll the victim toward the rescuer(s), keeping the neck in line with the rest of the back vertebrae. The backboard is then brought forward and slipped under the patient. Note the tie-downs that have been placed under the backboard, and the rolled-up towel that will be positioned under the victim's neck.

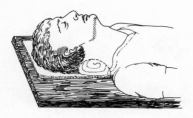

Details of proper neck support

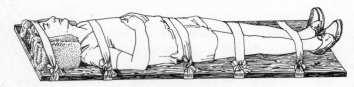

Place towels or pillows to support the head and neck and prevent any sideways movement. Strap the tie-downs together to completely immobilize the patient on the backboard.

For less severe injuries, such as neck or lower back strain, see below.

TREATMENT:

1. Use heat or cold on the affected area; either may help. Cold may be best for the first day or two. Be careful not to burn the patient with heat. Moist heat is better than a heating pad.
2. Encourage as much rest as possible until improvement is shown. In any case, rest is important; at times, absolute bed rest is necessary.
3. Avoid positions and movements that hurt, and activities that increase pain. Be patient. Pushing to return to normal activities too soon will delay final recovery.
4. Relax emotionally; tense muscles will delay recovery.
5. Massage sore muscles if it helps. Use firm but gentle massage; this "milks" the blood and helps to clear the soreness.
6. Stretch cramped muscles if injury is minor. Just as a "charley horse" in the calf hurts terribly until it is stretched, other muscles can also cramp, and will often respond to stretching in the same way.
7. Pain medication may be needed, but should be of moderate strength. In many cases, aspirin or Tylenol will suffice.

Note: The basic idea is that these kinds of minor injuries take time to clear. Anything that worsens the soreness should be avoided.

14.2 Bruises

Bruises must be differentiated from fractures. See section 14.4.

TREATMENT:

1. If available, ice should be applied immediately (one hour on and one hour off) to reduce swelling.
2. If ice is unavailable, seawater compresses should be applied in the same frequency as ice.

14.3 Sprains

A sprain is the stretching or tearing of a ligament. Sprains must be differentiated from fractures. See section 14.4. If you are not sure, it is safer to treat the injury as a fracture and splint and elevate it. Follow the directions for splinting, found in section 15.11.

TREATMENT: ("ICE"—Ice, Compression, Elevation)

1. If ice is available, apply intermittently for the first 48 hours to reduce swelling. If ice is not available, apply cool seawater compresses or soak affected area in a bucket or sink.
2. Sprained joints should be rested. Apply an Ace compression bandage or splint for at least ten days. See section 15.11.
3. If possible, do not walk if you have sprained an ankle or knee. Walking slows healing and prevents swelling from going down. It is much better to sit with the affected leg *elevated*.

14.4 Fractures

A fracture is any break in a bone. A simple or "closed" fracture is one in which the skin over the fracture site is not broken. A compound or "open" fracture is one in which the bone sticks through the skin or there is an open wound extending to or over the area of the broken bone. Fractures are seldom life-threatening, but they are very painful and can easily cause panic. *Slow down* and deal with them in the following manner.

First, be sure the injury is a fracture.

SIGNS AND SYMPTOMS:

1. Severe pain directly over the fracture site
2. An obvious deformity
3. Moderate to severe swelling
4. Discoloration (black and blue) around the site
5. A "grating" feeling, called *crepitus*, occurring when the bone ends rub together
6. If the fracture is "open," bone fragments may be seen.
7. Disability: Because of the pain, the person will refuse to use the affected limb or area.

Important Note: Not all of the signs of fracture may be present at the same time. If you suspect a fracture, but are not sure, treat the injury as a fracture until proven otherwise.

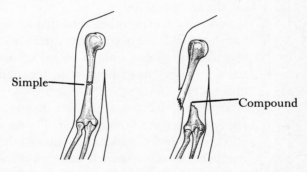

Simple and compound fractures (humerus bone of right arm)

TREATMENT OF A SIMPLE OR "CLOSED" FRACTURE:

1. Prior to splinting, an angulated (deformed) fracture should be straightened, or "reduced." If this is done immediately after the accident, little or no pain should occur.

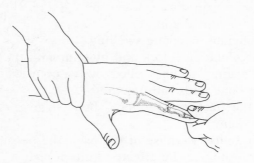

This general technique of reducing a fracture is also applicable to a dislocation. In the illustration, counter-traction is being applied at the wrist, while gentle traction is applied at the site of the deformity.

    a. First, gently cut or tear overlying clothing off the involved area.

    b. If another crew member is available, have him/her hold the extremity firmly above the fracture site. (This is called counter-traction.) With or without help, proceed as follows:

    c. Grasp the extremity with both hands and apply traction by pulling *gently*. Do *not* use hard, swift jerks, which may cause a bone fragment or ends of a bone to break through the skin, changing a previously simple fracture to a compound one.

    d. Hold on to your traction; do not let go until splinting is completed.

    e. If pain is severe, medication may be administered, such as Demerol, 50–75 mg IM. After the reduction, pain is to be expected, and an oral medication such as Tylenol #3 may be taken every 4 hours.

2. After the fracture is straightened, apply a splint that is long enough, well padded, and well secured to uninjured parts of the body. See section 15.11. *Remember:* Wrapping a splint too tightly may damage circulation in the involved extremity. If fingers or toes go numb, swell, or turn blue, the splint may be too tight. Loosen and reapply.

3. The splint should be kept on for 6 to 8 weeks (if no cast can be applied), to allow the bone to heal properly by not allowing movement of bony fragments or ends of bone.

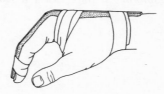

An aluminum splint with foam backing (if available) is applied as illustrated. Note the general shape the finger takes, as if a glass or cup is being grasped at the time the splint is applied.

COMMON FRACTURE SITES:

No attempt can be made in this context to list the treatment of every bone that could be fractured. *Remember:* Follow the general guidelines listed above and in section 15.11 for any fracture.

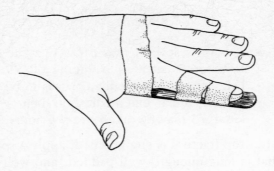

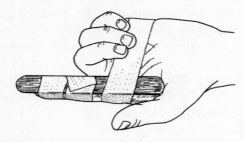

Another method of splinting a finger when a moldable splint is un-available.

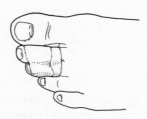

Tape the involved toe to one or more of the adjacent toes.

110

1. Finger

   These fractures will probably be among the most commonly encountered aboard, along with toe fractures, listed below. Treat a simple fracture with a marked deformity by gently pulling the end of the finger straight out while applying pressure on the deformity at the fracture site. This will align the bone ends in an approximate anatomical relationship. A splint is then applied to the top side of the finger. (See "Dislocations," section 14.5, as well as section 15.11.) Wear the splint for 6 weeks to allow for complete bone healing.

2. Toes

   If a marked deformity exists, reduction of the fracture is accomplished in the way mentioned above in finger fractures. Whether a deformity exists or not, simply tape (any kind of tape will do) the involved toe to the adjacent toe(s) for 6 weeks.

3. Nose

   Although the nose may be crooked, the only thing that needs immediate attention is control of the bleeding. See section 4.1.

4. Collarbone

   Apply figure-eight splint or Ace bandage if one is available. If not, put arm on injured side in a sling. This will reduce the pressure on the collarbone.

5. Wrist

   Position the arm so that there is a 90-degree bend at the elbow. Apply gentle traction by pulling up on fingers while another person (if available) grasps the arm just above the elbow and applies countertraction downward. Firm pres-

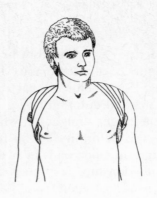

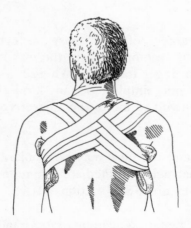

A typical figure-8 splint. Note the padding placed in the armpit region. This prevents injury from excessive pressure on vital nerves and blood vessels in the area.

sure at the site of deformity should move the bones back into place. A splint must be applied before letting go of the hand and wrist.

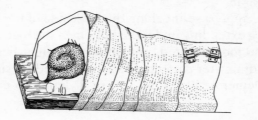

Details of proper immobilization of the wrist. The hand is grasping a rolled-up washcloth. A board, or other firm material, is placed under the wrist and extends to the mid-forearm. An Ace bandage, or other material, is wrapped firmly—but not too tightly—around the entire area, leaving the fingers free for visual inspection and gentle movement.

6. Ribs

Control the pain from a rib fracture by giving an oral pain medication, such as Tylenol #3, one every 4 hours; or if pain is severe, Demerol, 50–75 mg IM. It is not necessary to reduce (straighten) the fracture. The arm on the injured side may be splinted to the body and put in a sling. Taping is not necessary as this restricts lung expansion. One hopes that the broken rib end has not damaged a blood vessel or, more rarely seen, protruded inward and punctured a lung. The discussion of these complications is beyond the scope of this text.

7. Pelvis and hip

These are severe injuries, and the injured person should remain in bed in a flat position. Encourage fluid intake. Control pain with medication, such as Demerol, 75–100 mg IM.

A urethral catheter may have to be passed into the bladder to allow urine to pass. Refer to section 15.7.

8. Ankle

Apply a splint along the back side of the lower leg extending under the bottom of the foot. Keep the foot elevated, and allow no weight-bearing. Administer pain medications as needed, such as Demerol, 50–75 mg IM, or Tylenol #3 orally.

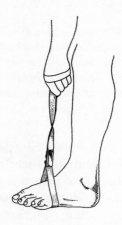

Prior to applying a figure-8 Ace bandage to the ankle, the foot should be flexed toward the head at a 90 degree angle. This is done voluntarily, or by using a sling of sorts to pull the toes upward.

TREATMENT OF A COMPOUND OR "OPEN" FRACTURE:

The object of treatment is to properly clean and protect from infection the bony ends protruding from the skin, and then straighten or "reduce" the fracture in the same manner as a simple fracture.

To begin with, pain medication will probably be required, such as Demerol, 50–100 mg IM. Then, proceed as follows:

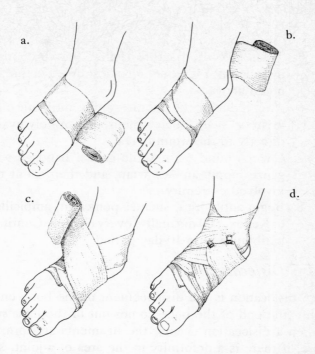

a. b.

c. d.

The Ace bandage is applied in a figure-8 in front of and behind the ankle joint. Wrap firmly, but not too tightly. If the toes become numb, start to tingle, or turn blue, the bandage is too tight and should be loosened.

1. Shave the area, taking care not to get any hair into the fracture site.
2. Use PhisoHex and sterile water (fresh water boiled for 20 minutes and then cooled) to scrub the area around the wound.
3. Remove any debris (dirt, tiny bone fragments) from the inner edges of the wound and clean area using sterile gauze.
4. Rinse inner edges with sterile water and clean again. After rinsing several more times with sterile water, realignment of the fracture may be attempted.

115

5. To reduce the fracture, follow the appropriate instructions for reduction of a simple fracture, as noted above.
6. After reducing the fracture, apply antibiotic ointment or cream, such as neosporin or Polymyxin, directly to the wound area.
7. Cover wound with sterile gauze; bandage with gauze, apply an Ace wrap, and then splint the involved extremity.
8. Begin antibiotics, such as penicillin, ampicillin, or Keflex, 500 mg orally, every 6 hours. Continue antibiotics for a 10-day period.

14.5 Dislocations

A dislocation is the displacement of the bone ends at a joint (the end of the bone comes out of the joint socket). When a dislocation occurs, the ligaments are torn; therefore, if there is a deformity in the area of a joint, suspect a dislocation. Sprains will not cause a deformity, but a dislocation *and* a fracture may occur together. The treatment of several commonly encountered dislocations is discussed below. In addition, refer to section 15.11.

1. Finger Dislocations
    a. Pull the end of the finger gently but firmly straight out until the bone is felt to "pop" back into the joint and the deformity disappears.
    b. Apply a splint to the top side of the finger with the finger in the "neutral" position. (When the arm is hanging straight down at the side of the body and the hand is relaxed, the fingers will assume a natural, flexed curve, referred to as the "neutral" position.)

2. Shoulder Dislocation

Severe pain may be present, and the affected side may appear lower than the other side.

   a. Administer pain medication, such as Demerol, 50–75 mg IM.

   b. Position the patient lying facedown on an elevated surface (upper bunk, cabin top, etc.), with the affected arm hanging straight down.

   c. Tie together (or put into a bucket) 10–15 pounds of weight and tie these to the patient's wrist on the affected side. *Protect* the wrist from rope burn and circulation impairment by *padding* the area generously before tying on the weights. As the muscles of the affected shoulder gradually tire out and the spasm decreases, the dislocation should correct. This will, at times, take up to an hour.

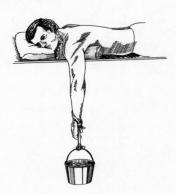

It is very important to place adequate padding under the armpit and around the wrist areas. The weights are then tied to the padded area. Make sure that no slippage occurs, as this would put unwanted pressure on the hand.

117

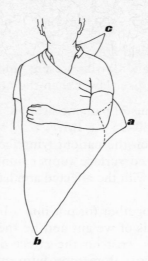

Any triangular piece of material can be formed into a sling. Point "A" is brought over in front of the elbow. Point "B" is then brought up and attached (by a pin or knot) to point "C," which has come from behind the back.

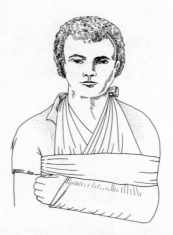

A "sling and swathe" is the addition of a bandage around the patient's chest and involved arm. This helps support the arm and immobilize it. The swathe is applied after the sling is in the proper position.

d. Apply a sling to the arm with the hand pointing at the opposite shoulder. The sling should be worn for 2 to 3 weeks.

3. Kneecap (patella) Dislocation

Many times, an audible "snap" or "pop" will occur, and the dislocation can be felt, usually just above the knee joint.

a. At times, the reduction can be accomplished quickly, without the need for pain medication.

b. Place one hand on the uppermost portion of the kneecap and push it toward the knee joint, at the same time extending the lower leg in a straight line by gently pulling on the lower part of the leg or ankle.

c. With the kneecap back in place, wrap the knee in an Ace bandage and apply a splint. Refer to section 15.11.

d. The affected leg should not be walked on for 2 to 3 weeks.

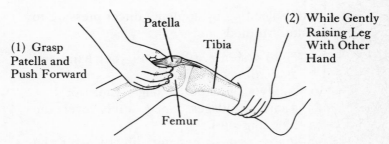

Reducing a superior dislocation of the patella

4. Toe Dislocations
   These are treated in the same way as finger dislocations.

   a. Pull the end of the toe gently but firmly out until the bone is felt to "pop" back into the joint and the deformity disappears.
   b. Tape the affected toe to the adjacent toe(s) for a period of 2 to 3 weeks.

14.6 Wounds

First, several definitions are in order:

Abrasion: Scraped skin, wound is superficial in nature
Laceration: Smooth or jagged cut, may be superficial or deep
Avulsion: A piece of skin is torn off or left hanging as a flap
Puncture: From nails, splinters, tips of knives, etc.
Crush: Injuries resulting in severely damaged tissue, which is usually grossly contaminated

IMMEDIATE TREATMENT OF ALL WOUNDS:

1. Control bleeding by applying direct pressure to the site. Methods are:

   a. Hold a sterile dressing in your hand and apply direct pressure.
   b. Apply a pressure bandage (gauze or 4 × 4-inch bandages taped firmly over the bleeding site).
   c. Place your bare hand directly over the bleeding site and apply pressure. Refer to section 2.3, "Bleeding and Shock."

2. Prevent contamination and infection from hair,

120

dirt, or other foreign bodies. This is also discussed in section 3.5b, "Wound Infections."

3. Determine whether the wound is superficial or deep by observation and gentle inspection. Deep wounds may cause damage to blood vessels, nerves, or tendons, and may result in disfigurement or disability. In general, no attempt to repair lacerated tendons or nerves should be made. However, if you see bleeding originating from a specific torn artery or vein, it may be necessary to tie off the very end of the vessel with a suture to prevent excessive bleeding. Refer to section 2.3, "Bleeding and Shock," and section 15.8, "Suturing—How to Close a Laceration."

TREATMENT OF ABRASIONS:

1. For bleeding abrasions, apply direct pressure over the bleeding area with a clean pad (towel, sheet, 4×4's, etc.) until the bleeding slows down or stops.
2. Clean the wound; mild bleeding may occur during cleansing. Use PhisoHex or soapy water (Ivory soap does nicely). Try to get dirt and any other debris out of the wound area; a sponge may be used to gently scrub the area.
3. When clean, apply an antibiotic cream or ointment, such as neosporin or Polymyxin.
4. Cover the area with a Telfa or adaptic pad, followed by gauze, which is wrapped around or taped over the affected area. These dressings may be changed twice daily if supplies permit.
5. If signs of wound infection are present, follow directions under section 3.5b, "Wound Infections."

TREATMENT OF SUPERFICIAL LACERATIONS:

1. Cleanse the area thoroughly, using PhisoHex or soapy water. Dry the area with sterile gauze.
2. Apply Steri-strips or butterfly tape bandages with slight tension; this is done by pulling the wound edges together before placing the strip bandages. The entire wound area should be covered with Steri-strips, which should be left in place for about 2 weeks. The area must be kept clean and dry.
3. Apply a bandage over everything. Change this bandage every day or so in order to check for wound infection.

TREATMENT OF DEEP LACERATIONS:

This is covered in section 15.8, "Suturing—How to Close a Laceration."

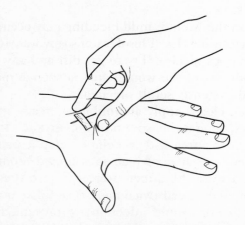

Steri-strip or butterfly Band-Aid application

Trauma

TREATMENT OF AVULSIONS:

Essentially, this is similar to the treatment of abrasions and superficial lacerations. If a skin flap is present, it may be gently placed back over the wound area after it has been thoroughly cleansed.

TREATMENT OF PUNCTURE WOUNDS:

Tetanus toxoid boosters should be up-to-date for all crew members. See "Immunizations," section 1.2.

1. Most puncture wounds need only to be cleansed well, then covered with an antibiotic cream or ointment such as neosporin or Polymyxin.
2. *Do not* go digging in a puncture wound for tiny pieces of glass or metal. These will frequently form a capsule around themselves, and can either work their way to a point directly below the surface of the skin, where they can be grabbed by forceps, or remain harmlessly where they are for many years. Trying to find a broken needle point or a glass fragment in the foot (or any other area) is often a time-consuming, painful, and frustrating experience, so leave them alone.
3. If signs of wound infection appear, refer to section 3.5b for treatment.

TREATMENT OF CRUSH INJURIES:

1. Cleanse the area thoroughly with PhisoHex or soapy water. This is a most important procedure, and should be done slowly and with care.
2. If a small area of mangled tissue is present, it can be cut off with scissors. Usually, there will be no pain sensation in the crushed tissue. However, if local anesthesia is necessary, refer to

section 15.8, "Suturing—How to Close a Laceration," which will give details about local anesthetic administration.

3. Suture, if necessary, following the instructions in section 15.8. Most of these injuries will heal whether they are stitched or not, but scarring will generally be somewhat more unsightly without suturing.

4. Apply an antibiotic cream or ointment, such as Polymyxin or neosporin.

5. In extensive crush injuries, administer oral antibiotics, such as penicillin, ampicillin, or Keflex, 250 mg every 6 hours for 10 days.

15. Procedures

15.1 Intravenous (IV) Fluids—Why and When to Administer

Intravenous fluids are used to replenish the body's supply of water and electrolytes, as well as calories and protein, in patients unable to tolerate oral fluids and food. They are also used to administer medications in patients unable to tolerate oral intake.

The question of how much IV fluid is required is a difficult one to answer. Not the least of our problems is that most vessels will not be carrying several bags of IV fluids. However, if supplies are obtainable, this section will assist you when you must make the decision to administer IV fluids.

Note: Water and electrolyte requirements should be met orally if at all possible. Soups (broths) and fruit juices (especially apple) can be given in small quantities at frequent intervals. Refer to section 5.2 for more specific diet suggestions. However, in situations where oral intake is not possible, IV's must be used to replace lost body fluids. Since a healthy person will begin showing signs of dehydration after several days without water intake, *consider IV fluid replacement in the following cases:*

1. Unconsciousness beyond 24–36 hours
2. Severe vomiting and diarrhea beyond 24–36 hours
3. Any situation where severe dehydration has already occurred, as in life-raft survivors, or in victims of severe heatstroke
4. The very ill person with a high fever who has no desire, is unable, or refuses to take oral fluids
5. Hemorrhage: This is covered in section 2.3, "Bleeding and Shock."

Generally, we need 2–3 liters of fluids, along with 5 grams of salt intake, every 24 hours to make up for the fluids lost through urination and sweating. In IV treatment, 2 liters of 5% dextrose and one liter of Ringer's lactate solution are used for this purpose. If fluid intake is still inadequate, or if increased loss of body fluids occurs, as in very hot weather or with severe vomiting or diarrhea, fluid requirements increase. In these cases, increased amounts of 5% dextrose and Ringer's lactate solution should be given.

How do you know if the body is getting enough fluids? *Urinary output* is probably your best guide. A healthy individual with good kidney function will put out approximately 40 cc of urine per hour, or 1000 cc in 24 hours. Use that as a rough guide. If less than 1000 cc per 24 hours is collected, more oral or IV fluids are required; if more than 1000 cc per 24 hours is collected, too much fluid is being given. These are, of course, rough guidelines. To complicate matters further, anyone who has heart or kidney problems will probably have special fluid requirements, but that discussion is beyond our scope.

A very accurate log of the patient's intake of oral and IV fluids, urinary output, blood pressure, and pulse should be recorded, every hour for the first 4 hours, then every 2–4 hours thereafter.

15.2 Intravenous (IV) Fluids—How to Start an IV

EQUIPMENT NEEDED:

1. Tourniquet
2. Alcohol
3. Butterfly needle
4. IV bottle (plastic) and tubing
5. Splint and tape for arm or hand

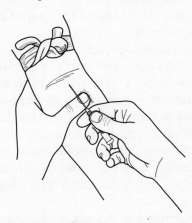

IV set-up: Note the tourniquet around the upper arm. Traction is placed on the skin below the site of the needle's insertion. The angle of the needle to the skin is about 45 degrees.

PROCEDURE:

1. Wash your hands thoroughly.
2. Attach the IV tubing to the IV bottle and flush the tubing so that fluid comes out the end of it.
3. Select a vein (veins do not pulsate) on top of the hand or in the crease of the elbow region.
4. Apply a tourniquet immediately above the selected site.
5. Cleanse the area with alcohol.
6. Apply tension on the skin below the site of insertion.
7. Insert the needle (do *not* touch it to anything else) at about a 45-degree angle to the skin, into the center of the vein. A backflow of blood into the syringe or tubing will indicate satisfactory placement.
8. Attach the IV tubing to the end of the needle housing or tubing.
9. Release the tourniquet.
10. Adjust the clamp and start the IV fluid running at a slow drip. The bottle is calibrated in cc's or milliliters, so you will know the rate at which the fluid is running out of the bottle.
11. If swelling occurs immediately, the needle is not in the vein; the infusion should be stopped, the needle removed, and the insertion site bandaged. Begin the entire procedure again at a different site.
12. If no swelling occurs, apply antibiotic cream or ointment, such as neosporin or Polymyxin.
13. Tape the needle firmly to the skin.
14. Cover the area with sterile 4-×-4-inch bandages, and secure with tape.

Procedures

15. Put an armboard or splint under the person's arm for support, and tape the arm to it.
16. *Log the date, time, insertion site, and contents of the IV infusion.*

15.3 Intramuscular (IM) Injections—How to Give Them

An IM injection is used when taking oral medications will be unsuccessful for a variety of reasons, including nausea and vomiting, unconsciousness, severe pain, or an uncooperative patient.

EQUIPMENT NEEDED:

1. Sterile syringe—2–3 cc will do nicely
2. Sterile needle, preferably 21-gauge
3. PhisoHex or betadine
4. Alcohol
5. Medication in a sterile ampule or vial

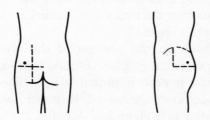

Intramuscular injection site (buttocks)

PROCEDURE:

1. Have the patient sit or lie down.
2. Cleanse the area to be injected with PhisoHex or betadine, then remove these agents with alcohol.

129

3. Attach the base of the needle to the syringe (if it isn't already).
4. Cleanse the top of the medicine bottle with alcohol, or break the ampule at its neck, being careful not to cut yourself or spill the contents.
5. Invert the bottle, insert the needle into its rubber top, and inject several cc's of air. This will allow the medication to be drawn more easily into the syringe. Injecting air is unnecessary when medication is drawn from an ampule.
6. Draw the appropriate amount of medication into the syringe, which is calibrated for measurement. Then remove the needle from the bottle or ampule.
7. Point the syringe and needle upward and tap on the syringe several times. Then, gently expel any air or bubbles in it by slowly pushing on the plunger until a drop of medicine appears at the needle tip.
8. Grasp the area around the injection site, without touching the actual site, and insert the needle at a steep angle.
9. Pull back on the plunger of the syringe and make sure that no blood enters. If blood is present, the needle is probably in a blood vessel and needs to be removed. Reinsert into another area after first cleansing the site.
10. Inject the medication slowly and evenly.
11. Gently withdraw the needle.
12. Keep the patient sitting or lying down for at least 10–15 minutes before letting him/her move around.

PRECAUTIONS:

1. Sterile technique must be maintained.

2. Double-check the medication and dosage you are using.
3. Be sure to remove the needle if you enter a blood vessel. The injection should be IM, not IV.

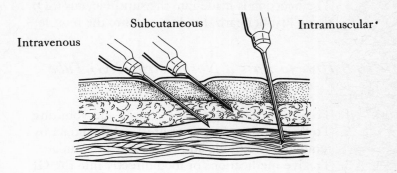

Illustration of the angle of the needle and relative depth when puncturing skin.

4. Nerves or tendons may be injured if careless technique is used or if an improper site is chosen. If a nerve is hit, there is usually a tingling sensation in the immediate area or somewhere in the extremity. Remove the needle and choose a different site.

15.4 Subcutaneous (SQ) Injections—How to Give Them

EQUIPMENT:

1. 25-gauge needle, ¾-inch long
2. 2-cc syringe
3. Medication (usually epinephrine, 1:1000 solution)

PROCEDURE:

1. Follow steps 1–7 listed in section 15.3 under IM injections.
2. Hold the needle at a 45-degree angle to the skin.
3. The injection is made into the subcutaneous (SQ) tissue just beneath the skin, *not* into the muscle.

15.5 How to Pass a Nasogastric (NG) Tube

WHY:

1. To prevent or help relieve nausea and vomiting
2. To decompress the gastrointestinal (GI) tract by removing the fluids and gases that accumulate
3. To give medications or food directly into the GI tract

EQUIPMENT NEEDED:

1. A nasogastric (NG) tube, size 16 or 18 French
2. A glass of water
3. Tape
4. Vaseline
5. Basin for stomach contents or vomitus

GENERALITIES:

The insertion of a nasogastric tube for gastric suctioning or tube feeding can be a perilous procedure. Note the following *if*'s:

1. If the patient chokes or gags violently, the tube has probably been inserted down his windpipe (trachea) instead of his esophagus. Remove the tube immediately.
2. If too much tube is inserted into the stomach, the end of the tube can curl around itself in a

knot and prevent both its easy removal and its effective use.

3. If not enough tube is inserted, gastric drainage will not be effective, since the end of the tube has to be in the stomach.

4. If force is used during insertion, a nosebleed can occur. Gently remove the tube and follow directions for "Nosebleed," section 4.1.

Most people will gag, fight, and generally not enjoy this procedure, so carefully explain what you are doing and why. Gentle but firm advancement of the tube will usually achieve success at the first try.

PROCEDURE:

1. The patient should be sitting upright if possible, or be on his side if lying down.

2. Lubricate the tip of the NG tube with Vaseline. The tip is the one with holes in it.

3. Insert the tip *gently* into one nostril and advance the tube downward and backward until the patient feels it reach the back of his throat.

4. If you are unable to pass the tube down one nostril because of blockage (this is very common), try the other one.

5. Ask the patient to swallow some water. As he/she is swallowing, advance the tube into the stomach. *If gagging is severe, or coughing or gasping for breath occurs, remove the tube and start again.*

6. Usually, if adequately lubricated, the tube can be passed in a matter of 30–45 seconds.

7. The tube should have black markings on it to indicate how much to pass. Be careful not to insert too much tube, as it can knot around itself and create additional problems.

8. When the tube is in place, the stomach contents can then be suctioned out by a bulb syringe, or the tube can be allowed to drain spontaneously.
9. If the tube blocks up, put an ounce or two of water down it to clear the plugged end.
10. Tape the tube to the side of the patient's face.
11. Apply Vaseline to the nasal area to keep the mucosa moist.
12. Rotate the tube every day to prevent it from sticking to one area of the stomach lining.

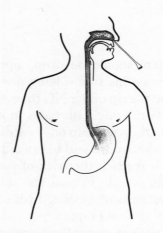

Nasogastric tube: The N/G tube is passed through the nose, down the esophagus, and into the stomach.

15.6 Nasogastric (NG) Feeding—When and What

WHEN:

Since for most previously healthy people, solid food is not needed to sustain life for at least four or five days, tube-feeding should be avoided if there's a reasonable expectation that professional medical help can be reached within that time. Tube-feeding is *not* something to be undertaken lightly or with undue haste. However, if under the verbal direction of a physician, or if circumstances permit no alternatives, then the following guidelines may be used in the attempt to keep someone alive until further medical treatment can be obtained.

Note: First, be sure the NG tube has been passed properly. See section 15.5.

WHAT:

Food must be puréed in order to pass through the NG tube. "Puréed" means ground, mashed, and blended until it is the consistency of baby food. (Naturally, you can use baby food if you already have it available.)

The object is to provide approximately one calorie per milliliter of a nutritionally balanced mixture over a time period of 24 hours. This should work out to 1800 calories in 1800 milliliters in 24 hours.

PROCEDURE:

1. Wash hands and kitchen utensils thoroughly.
2. Use utensils to remove food from jars or cans. Try to avoid touching the food with your hands.
3. Thoroughly clean a container that holds at least 8 cups. Seven and one-half cups of puréed food from the following list will provide the 1800 calories to be administered in 24 hours. You can choose the type of meat, vegetable, and fruit from the list of substitutes provided.
4. Place all the food in the container and add water up to the 7½-cup level.
5. Purée. Since you will probably not have a blender

135

aboard, you'll have to chop, mash, stir, and, if possible, pressure-cook all the food until the mixture is the consistency of baby food.

6. Use a syringe to transfer the puréed food into the NG tube.
7. Keep the mixture refrigerated or cooled, and use it all within a 24-hour period. Three hundred milliliters, or approximately 1½ cups of the mixture, can be given every 4 hours; or give five feedings a day, until the 7½ cups are gone.

The following example will provide an 1800-calorie, 1800-milliliter mixture:

Puréed meat—2 jars (7½-oz size)
Egg—one
Puréed vegetable—2 jars (7½-oz size)
Strained fruit—2 jars
Evaporated milk—1 can (13-oz size)
Skim milk powder—⅓ can (13-oz size)
Orange juice—½ can (13-oz size)
Bread without crusts—4 slices
Margarine—1 teaspoon
Water—to bring total of container up to 7½ cups

The above combination will provide approximately 107.6 grams of protein, 60.8 grams of fat, and 219.4 grams of carbohydrate, and will equal about 1800 calories, or one calorie per milliliter of mixture.

SUGGESTED FOODS AND SUB-
STITUTES
BEVERAGES:
milk, buttermilk, milk shakes, malts, cocoa

FOODS TO AVOID

coffee and caffeinated beverages, carbonated and alcoholic beverages

Procedures

BREADS & CEREALS:
toast and crackers

untoasted bread, crusts, hot breads, waffles, pancakes, rolls, doughnuts, dry cereals

MEATS & SUBSTITUTES:
beef, veal, lamb, chicken, turkey, pork, cottage cheese, yogurt, American cheese

crisp, coarse, tough, whole or ground dry meat or fish or poultry. Hard cheese, bacon, sausage.

EGGS:
poached, boiled, scrambled

fried eggs

POTATOES & SUBSTITUTES:
white potatoes, sweet potatoes, macaroni, noodles, spaghetti

all others

VEGETABLES:
puréed cooked vegetables, tomato juice

all others, including gassy vegetables, such as cauliflower, broccoli, cabbage, etc.

FRUITS:
puréed canned fruit, ripe bananas, all fruit juices

whole or fresh fruit, except bananas

FATS:
butter or margarine, cream, half and half, whipping cream, sour cream, mayonnaise

bacon, nuts, avocado, peanut butter, fried foods

SOUPS:
cream or broth soups (strained)

soups made with chunks of food

DESSERTS:
custard, simple pudding such as vanilla, tapioca, cornstarch; flavored gelatin, plain ice cream or sherbert.

pie, any dessert containing nuts, seeds, skins, or pieces of fruit. All other cakes and cookies

SWEETS & CONDIMENTS:
as desired, mild seasoning, herbs and spices, sugar, salt, honey, clear jelly, syrup

pickles, olives, nuts

I know all of this is confusing. My suggestion is that if you're sure you'll have to tube-feed someone, then reread this section, try to get a good idea of what you will be doing, then just do it. Remember, this is a last-resort measure for someone who can't or won't eat for five days or so. *Don't* rush into it if you're going to reach port in the very near future. Needless to say, obtain medical assistance as soon as possible.

15.7 *Bladder Catheterization—How to Do It*

WHY:

1. A catheter is used to allow the bladder to empty in patients who are unconscious, or otherwise unable to urinate in a normal way.
2. Urinary output serves as a guide in determining how much IV fluid a patient will require.

EQUIPMENT NEEDED:

1. A sterile catheter set contains all that is required: i.e., sterile gloves, lubricant, a disposable catheter (a #16 or 18 French Foley catheter is adequate for adults), and a collection bag.

PROCEDURE:

1. If the patient is conscious, explain the procedure calmly to reassure him/her.
2. Try to keep the immediate area and all items sterile; be careful about touching anything not involved in the procedure.
3. Put on sterile gloves.
4. Lubricate the end of the catheter and proceed as follows:

Males:

5. Cleanse the end of the penis with the betadine solution supplied in the kit. Repeat.
6. Gently grasp the penis and hold it straight up as you insert the end of the catheter into the urethra (this is the canal from the bladder to the end of the penis).
7. Advance the catheter to where it bifurcates (turns into two exits) or until urine flows freely.

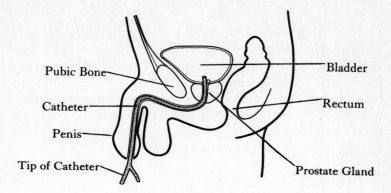

Bladder catheterization

Females:

5. Separate the labia in order to see the urethral opening.
6. Cleanse the area with betadine, wiping downward. Repeat.
7. Insert the catheter 2–3 inches into the urethra, at which point urine should begin to flow.

Males and Females:

8. Urine *must* be flowing before you inflate the balloon at the end of the catheter, which you do by following the directions on the kit. Return of urine is very important before proceeding.
9. Connect the catheter to the collection bag.
10. Tape the catheter to the patient's thigh.
11. Wash and cleanse (with PhisoHex or betadine) the area where the catheter enters the urethra at least once daily.
12. Drain the collection bag every 8 hours and *record in the log* how many cc's of urine were in the bag (the bag should be marked in cc's).

Note: Ideally, the above should be performed in a sterile manner. However, given the confines of a vessel and less than optimum working conditions, I would suggest that an antibiotic be administered to the patient, if one is not already being given. Refer to the treatment of urinary-tract infections, section 3.4a. A Foley catheter can be left in place for 5–7 days, after which time the incidence of infection rises, so antibiotics are advised.

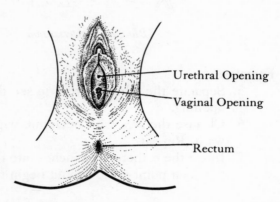

Bladder catheterization

15.8 Suturing—How to Close a Laceration

EQUIPMENT:

1. Prepackaged three-piece suture set. This set contains a needle holder, tissue forceps, and scissors. These instruments are reusable. They are sterile when packaged; after the first use they must be resterilized. See section 15.9.
2. Prepackaged suture (thread). Many sizes and types are available, but a 3-0 or 4-0 ethilon or silk suture is satisfactory for most needs. (I use eth-

ilon most frequently in the emergency department.)

3. A 5-cc or 10-cc syringe with a 23-gauge needle (all prepackaged) for administering the local anesthetic. A plastic syringe cannot be resterilized in boiling water. Either carry more than one or use a glass syringe, which can be boiled.
4. Xylocaine, 1% plain. This local anesthetic is available in 50-cc bottles.
5. An antibiotic cream or ointment (such as neosporin).
6. Bandages.

PROCEDURE:

1. Clean the area well, using PhisoHex and sterile water. See instructions under "Abrasions," section 14.6.
2. Apply the local anesthetic to the wound area:

   a. Draw 5–10 cc of 1% xylocaine plain into the syringe and inject this subcutaneously into the wound edges all along the length of the laceration (both sides).
   b. If more xylocaine is needed, be sure to put a new needle on the syringe before drawing more xylocaine out of the bottle. If a used needle is inserted into the bottle to draw more xylocaine, the contents of the bottle will be contaminated.

3. Wait 10–15 minutes after injecting the local anesthetic for the maximum effect to occur. The wound area will have no sensation at that time, which will enable you to proceed with no discomfort to the patient.
4. Suture the wound:

141

a. Grasp the needle in the middle by the needle holder.
b. Use the tissue forceps to gently grasp one side of the laceration and turn the edge upward.
c. Push the needle through one side of the cut and then the other side.
d. Continue in one of two ways:

1. Running stitch:
   —Pull the suture until about one inch remains visible and put a knot in that end.
   —Lay the suture over the top of the skin edges in the direction of the opposite end of the laceration and about 1/4–1/3 inch down the line, and repeat step c above.
   —At the last stitch, which is at the end of the laceration, put another knot in the end and cut off the suture, leaving about 1/2 inch after the knot.

2. Individual stitch:
   —Tie a square knot, which will pull the edges gently together.
   —Cut the ends, leaving about 1/2 inch above the knot.

Remember: The skin edges should come together gently. Do *not* pull them together so hard that the tissue is caved upward and looks "squashed."

142

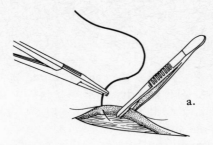

a.

The needle is gripped in the middle of its curve. Skin is retracted with forceps. For both simple and running stitches, the skin edges are brought together gently, not squeezed tightly by the stitch.

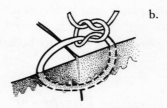

b.

Simple stitch: An individual square knot is made.

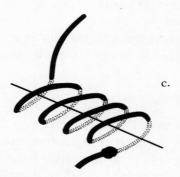

c.

Running stitch: An over, under, continuous stitch, which is knotted at both ends.

5. Cover the wound with antibiotic cream or ointment.
6. Apply bandages to the entire area. Keep the bandages clean and dry; if they get wet or dirty, change them. Otherwise, a dressing change every 2–3 days is sufficient.
7. Leave the sutures in place:
    Head and face—4–5 days
    Extremities—10–14 days
    Chest and back—7–10 days
8. To remove sutures, cut the individual sutures and pull them out. In the case of a running suture, cut one knot and gently but firmly pull the other end out. At times, several areas of the running stitch may have to be cut to ease its removal.

15.9 How to Sterilize Equipment

For glass syringes and needles:

1. Boil the item in water for 20 minutes, or in a pressure cooker under 15 pounds of pressure for 20 minutes.
2. Remove the items without contaminating them. Ideally, one sterile instrument is used to remove all others.

For metal instruments:

1. Boil as in step 1 above.
2. An alternative is to wash the item carefully, then place it briefly in alcohol, then light the alcohol. Allow the item to cool before using it.
3. Many items are supplied in sterile, disposable packages. They are not bulky, and may be the

best idea for long-term storage in dry, confined areas aboard. However, once used, these items must be discarded.

15.10 How to Remove Embedded Fish Hooks

1. *Do not* attempt to pull the hook out backward. Push the hook straight through in the direction of the barb. At times, local anesthetic may be necessary. Refer to section 15.8, procedure steps 1–3.
2. Clip off the barb with wire cutters.
3. Remove the remainder of the hook by pulling it out backwards.
4. Wash the area with PhisoHex or betadine.
5. Put an antibiotic cream or ointment (neosporin or Polymyxin) dressing over the wound.
6. If infection occurs, refer to section 4.5b.

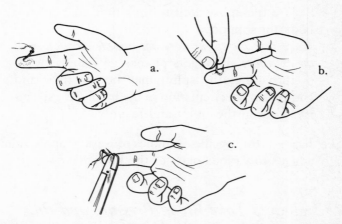

Fish hook removal: The hook is pushed straight through the skin in the direction of the barb, which is then clipped off with wire cutters. The remaining shank of the hook is then removed through the original puncture site.

15.11 Splinting and Bandaging—How to Do It

A splint can be made from any material (such as a bunk-board, pillow, piece of cardboard, a padded piece of scrap wood, etc.). Otherwise, an air splint or aluminum splint, along with Kling dressings, Band-Aids, and gauze 4 × 4's, should be available in the ship's medicine chest.

PROCEDURE:

1. Cover all open wounds with a sterile dressing. Elaborate bandaging techniques are unnecessary, but the bandage must be sterile to protect the wound from infection.
2. The splint should be padded (a pillow will work) to prevent pressure points and pain.
3. The splint should be long enough to extend just past the joints above and below the affected bony area.
4. Secure the splint well to uninjured parts of the body for support.
5. *Make sure the splint does not impede circulation of the extremity.* If fingers or toes go numb, swell, or turn blue, the splint may be too tight and could damage circulation in the involved extremity. Loosen the splint and reapply.

See diagrams for specific examples of ways to apply splints and bandages to various parts of the body.

15.12 How to Take Blood Pressure and Pulse

15.12a Blood Pressure

EQUIPMENT NEEDED:

1. Blood pressure cuff (sphygmomanometer—try

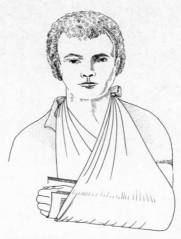

The wrist has been splinted using a magazine. A sling is then applied. Injuries of the elbow, forearm, wrist, or hand can be immobilized in much the same way.

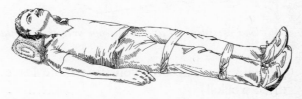

Immobilization of an injury of a lower extremity. Since a neck injury is not suspected, a pillow may be placed under the head and neck for comfort.

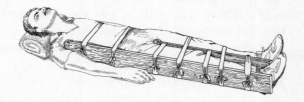

Splints, in this case of wood, are placed on both sides of the leg to immobilize the injured site. Note the padding in the armpit, groin, and ankle regions.

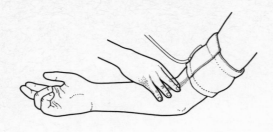

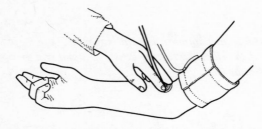

Location of blood pressure cuff and stethescope over the brachial artery

pronouncing that after your first shore leave in three weeks!)
2. Stethoscope

PROCEDURE:
1. Wrap the deflated blood-pressure cuff around the upper arm, about an inch above the crease of the elbow. This will be just above where the brachial artery will be felt and listened to.
2. The arm should be held at the level of the heart, whether the patient is sitting or lying down.
3. Keeping a finger (not your thumb) on the radial artery pulse at the wrist, and with the cuff valve shut down, inflate the cuff by squeezing the bulb to a level 30 mm of mercury above the level where you can't feel the radial pulse anymore.

The reading will be in mm of mercury on the gauge.

4. Place the end of the stethoscope over the brachial artery at the crease of the elbow, hold it there with your fingers (not your thumb), and put the earpieces in your ears.

5. *Slowly* deflate the cuff by releasing its valve. This will cause the pressure on the gauge to fall, and you will hear arterial pulsations through the stethoscope.

6. When you hear the first pulsation, note the reading on the gauge. This is the *systolic* pressure. As the pressure continues to be released (try to release it 2–3 mm of mercury at each pulsation), the pulse sounds will usually increase in intensity, then gradually decrease until they are no longer heard. At that point, again note the reading on the gauge. This is the *diastolic* pressure.

7. The blood pressure (BP) reading is written down as systolic/diastolic such as 120/80, 140/100, 100/70, etc.

8. There may be a great variety in blood pressure readings between different people. Furthermore, activity, emotional changes, age, the time of day, and, of course, illness, may affect the blood pressure. Generally, a *normal* adult blood pressure is somewhere about 100–140 mm mercury systolic over 60–90 mm mercury diastolic.

9. Always *record* your findings in the log, and note the time the blood pressure was taken. Try to use the same arm when you repeat a BP reading.

15.12b *Pulse*

SITES:

1. Radial artery (just inside the crease of the wrist)
2. Brachial artery (at the crease of the elbow)
3. Carotid artery (at the sides of the neck)
4. Femoral artery (in the groin area)
5. Directly over the heart

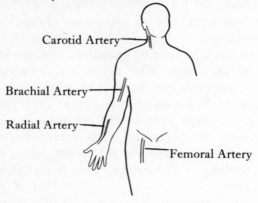

Location of arterial pulses

PROCEDURE:

1. Do *not* press too firmly on the artery; the vessel can be squeezed too tightly for a pulse to be felt.
2. Do *not* use your thumb. Use your index and/or middle finger.
3. Place your finger(s) lightly over the arterial pulsation at one of the sites listed above.
4. *Record* the number of beats per minute as the *pulse rate*. Average is 60–80 beats per minute in adults, but this can vary considerably with conditions, age, activity, etc.
5. *Record* whether the pulse is regular or not, and whether the force of the pulsations is strong or weak.

16. Dentistry at Sea

by Steve Scharf, D.D.S.

16.1 Introduction

Most common dental emergencies are preventable. Before an extended cruise, a thorough visual and X-ray exam can eliminate an inconvenient (at best) episode. If you tell your dentist that you won't be receiving dental care for an extended time, it may change his recommendations for your dental care.

A boat several weeks away from landfall is a poor excuse for a dental office, but there are things that can and should be done to ease a person's suffering. A "toothache," a "broken jaw," or a "swollen jaw" are not specific enough descriptions to begin treatment of a dental emergency. The first step is to evaluate the symptoms accurately and determine a diagnosis. The next step is to administer simple but effective treatment.

16.2 Toothache

16.2a Uncomplicated Toothache

Cause: Deep decay near the pulp of the tooth, or a broken tooth that exposes the pulp. "Uncomplicated" does not necessarily mean that it is easy to treat or that it hurts less than other types of toothache. It just means that the main symptom, spontaneous pain, is not accompanied by other symptoms, such as swelling or fever.

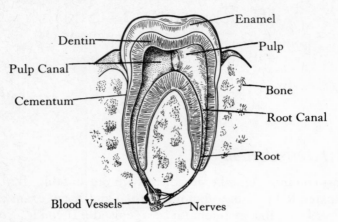

Anatomy of a tooth

SIGNS AND SYMPTOMS:

1. Pain only in the area of the affected tooth. The difference between this type of toothache and others is that the pulp of the tooth is alive, but it is very inflamed.
2. Test to see if this is an uncomplicated toothache: Place the coldest water available next to the tooth and it should hurt. Heat can be used as an alternative, but cold is best.

TREATMENT:

1. Identify the tooth.
2. Clean the debris from the area with a rinse of water or a piece of gauze.
3. Use dental tweezers to place a small piece of cotton saturated with oil of cloves or "toothache drops" directly over the affected area.

152

4. Relief will be temporary, and the treatment will need to be repeated fairly often.
5. Administer pain medication orally, such as Tylenol #3, one every 3–4 hours.
6. A dentist should be seen as soon as possible as the tooth is probably about to abscess.

16.2b Toothache Due to Dental Abscess

Cause: decay or trauma that has killed the pulp inside the tooth, and the pulp has now become infected.

SIGNS AND SYMPTOMS:

1. Pain, from mild to severe. It will occur by itself, although heat may make it worse.
2. Tooth may be very tender to biting and touch.
3. Swelling: from slight to severe. Look in the mouth around the tooth for swelling, as well as the face and neck. The tooth may or may not have an obvious area of decay.

TREATMENT:

1. Administer pain medication, such as Tylenol #3 orally, or Demerol 50–75 mg IM. Usually, only medication will provide relief of pain, although sometimes, the application of cold compresses may help. *Do not* place aspirin on the gum— aspirin destroys gum tissue.
2. Take the person's temperature and record it in the ship's log.
3. Administer a broad-spectrum antibiotic immediately, such as penicillin, ampicillin, or Keflex, 250–500 mg every 6 hours orally.
4. If the swelling is *worse* after two days, and the person shows signs of systemic illness, such as fever, lack of appetite, general aches, etc., the

abscess may have to be lanced (opened) with a scalpel.

   a. With a piece of gauze, hold the lip or cheek away from the gum to gain access to the swollen area.

   b. Feel the swollen area. All swelling will benefit from lancing. You *must* be able to identify a fluid-filled area. If the swollen area is firm and does not move with moderate pressure, *do not* lance it.

   c. Insert the tip of the scalpel into the center of the fluid-filled area. If no pus appears, try once again. *Do not* repeatedly stab the area; you may have been fooled into thinking a generalized swelling was fluid when it was not. Blood-letting is *not* an accepted treatment!

5. If swelling is increasing, the person is getting sicker, and you either could not find an area to drain, or were unsuccessful, get some very warm water and a clean cloth and begin applying moist heat on the outside of the face over the swollen area. This will increase the blood supply, which brings the body's natural defenses and the antibiotic to the area in greater strength, and should help bring the abscess to a head, usually on the skin surface.

   a. You can try to drain (lance) the abscess again, or the abscess may drain spontaneously where you applied the heat.

   b. *Do not* resort to this unless you are really worried about the person's deteriorating condition, as an abscess that drains through the skin will leave a scar. Of course, a facial scar is better than more dire consequences of infection, but it is to be avoided if possible.

16.2c Toothache Due to Gum Abscess (Periodontal Abscess)

CAUSE: periodontal (gum) disease, called *pyorrhea*, which is basically a destructive disease of the gum tissue and the bone around the teeth.

SIGNS AND SYMPTOMS:

1. Can be similar to dental abscess, as in section 16.2b, except usually less severe, and will often drain spontaneously into the tissue alongside the affected tooth.
2. Spontaneous pain (not caused by heat, cold, chewing, etc.), which is not relieved by anything except pain medication.
3. The tooth may be loose, and very tender to the touch.
4. Swelling, often confined to the area immediately around the tooth, although it can spread.

TREATMENT:

1. Hot saltwater rinses, using a solution of ½ teaspoonful of salt in 8 ounces of water. Instruct the person to fill their mouth with the solution and swish it around until the water cools. Repeat often.
2. Maintain brushing and flossing around the affected tooth. This may hurt, but it is necessary.
3. Administer a broad-spectrum antibiotic, such as penicillin, ampicillin, or Keflex, 250 mg orally every 6 hours, for 10–14 days.

4. Administer medication for pain, as needed, such as Tylenol #3 orally, one every 3–4 hours.

16.3 Dental Trauma

16.3a Bleeding

CAUSE: Since the mouth is provided with a generous blood supply, any wound, even relatively minor in nature, will tend to bleed profusely, especially lacerations of the tongue or lip.

TREATMENT:

1. Take several small pieces of gauze and apply moderate pressure to the bleeding area.
2. The bleeding should subside in 5–10 minutes, but will likely start again with little provocation.
3. See below, section 3.2.

16.3b Lacerations

CAUSE: as above, section 3.1

TREATMENT:

1. A small, clean wound, such as could occur when the tongue or lips are caught between the teeth when a blow to the chin is delivered, will require no treatment other than rinsing the mouth with plain water after meals, thereby keeping the area clean.
2. A larger wound, or one of any size which has debris implanted in it, should be cleansed with sterile water and 2 × 2-inch gauze pads. Use *lots* of water. If water is in short supply, a combination of water and betadine may be used to clean the wound. Use gauze to gently clean out the debris.

3. Most of the time, suturing inside the mouth will not be necessary, as the mucosa will heal by itself, along with the above treatment. Professional assistance will be necessary if the laceration inside the mouth is so large that the bleeding will not stop or healing will not take place.
4. Administer a broad-spectrum antibiotic, such as penicillin, ampicillin, or Keflex, 250 mg orally every 6 hours for 7–10 days, or until healing is complete.

16.3c Loose Teeth

TREATMENT:

1. Try to position a loose tooth by grasping hold of the tooth between your thumb and forefinger. A 2 × 2 gauze will increase your grip.
2. Loose teeth which do not require repositioning should be left alone. A dentist would splint them, but that is not practical at sea.
3. Diet should be restricted to soft or liquid foods, so as to not bear down chewing on the affected tooth.
4. Keep the area clean by frequent rinses of the mouth.

16.3d Missing Teeth

TREATMENT:

1. A permanent tooth which has been knocked out and is still in one piece can be replanted if it is done soon, preferably within 15–30 minutes.
2. *Do not* wash or scrub the tooth. The root is covered with delicate and important tissues. Rinse *gently* in plain water.
3. Place the tooth in its position, and have the pa-

tient hold it in place for 30–45 minutes. This maneuver is difficult for both the victim and the novice helper.

4. Administer a broad-spectrum antibiotic immediately, and continue for 10–14 days. Penicillin, ampicillin, or Keflex, 250–500 mg every 6 hours orally, may be given.
5. Obtain dental assistance as soon as possible, as a root canal may be required.

16.3e Broken Teeth

TREATMENT:

1. A small chip in a tooth is not cause for immediate concern, although it may be annoying and sharp to the tongue.
2. A moderate fracture of a tooth will result in exposed dentin and will be sensitive to hot, cold, and touch; but no treatment is required.
3. A severe fracture will expose the pulp (nerve) of the tooth and will cause a toothache. Furthermore, the pulp will be exposed to bacteria from the mouth, thereby possibly causing its destruction.
   a. Administer oral pain medication, such as Tylenol #3, as well as toothache drops, such as oil of cloves, for pain relief.
   b. As the pulp dies, it may cause an abscess. If any swelling occurs, administer an antibiotic, such as penicillin, ampicillin, or Keflex, 250–500 mg orally every 6 hours.

16.3f Broken Jaw

SIGNS AND SYMPTOMS:

1. May be indicated by teeth which no longer fit

together when attempting to bite, after a history of trauma to the area

2. There will probably be bruising and swelling of the area around the teeth and gums.
3. Pain will be present upon movement of the jaw or when attempting to chew.

TREATMENT:

1. Administer pain medication if necessary, such as Tylenol #3 orally, or Demerol, 50–75 mg IM.
2. Restrain the jaw from moving. Gently wrap an elastic bandage around the top and back of the head and around the chin.
3. Administer antibiotics, orally if possible, such as penicillin, ampicillin, or Keflex, 250 mg every 6 hours.
4. A liquid or very soft diet will be necessary.
5. Obtain dental assistance when available.

16.4 Oral Hygiene

16.4a Herpes ("fever blisters"); Aphthous ulcers

SIGNS AND SYMPTOMS:

1. One, or many, sores throughout the mouth or on the lips.
2. Pain in the area of the sores; may be quite severe.

TREATMENT:

1. There is no proven effective treatment which shortens the duration of the disease. Treatment is aimed at preventing complications and easing suffering.
2. Good nutrition, especially fluids, is essential, particularly if the patient is refusing to eat because of the discomfort of the sores.

3. Keep the area clean of food debris by gently and thoroughly rinsing with plain water.
4. Usually, the sores will go away by themselves in about 10–14 days. Antibiotics are *not* required.

16.4b Trench Mouth

CAUSE: Caused by a specific bacterium in susceptible people. Can cause some permanent damage to the gum tissue.

SIGNS AND SYMPTOMS:
1. Discomfort
2. Unpleasant smell to the breath
3. The gum tissue looks awful; it may be abscessed, with reddish-yellow areas between the teeth.

TREATMENT:
1. Administer a broad-spectrum antibiotic, such as penicillin, ampicillin, Keflex, or erythromycin, 250 mg orally every 6 hours for 10–14 days.
2. Cleanse the teeth *several times a day* with a toothbrush and floss. Cleaning will cause discomfort and bleeding, but it must be done. Softening the bristles of a nylon toothbrush in hot water for a few seconds before brushing will ease the pain of brushing.
3. Good nutrition and vitamin intake is to be encouraged.

16.5 Emergency Dental Kit

1. Dental mouth mirror; inexpensive ones are for sale at some drugstores, or ask your dentist to sell you one.
2. Small flashlight or penlight

3. Cotton pliers, a type of tweezer for placing and removing small items. Referred to in treatment instructions as "tweezers"
4. Several tongue blades; to retract the cheek and tongue
5. 2 × 2-inch gauze pads, sterilized and wrapped; used to clean oral wounds and to hold onto the tongue, lips, or teeth
6. Clean cotton; to apply toothache drops
7. Toothache drops; oil of cloves is the classic medication, but other preparations are available; "Eugenol" is the active ingredient.
8. Betadine; for cleansing oral wounds
9. Scalpel, with sterile blade; a #11 or #15 will suffice
10. Pain medication, such as Tylenol #3 for oral use or Demerol for IM injections

Appendix 1

Comprehensive Emergency Medical Kits

I have been asked to organize the "ship's medicine chest" in a variety of vessels, both pleasure and commercial. The most common question I am asked is "What do I need in my medical kit?" After a discussion of individual requirements, the contents of a kit are decided upon, based upon the following general guidelines:

1. The size of the vessel (How much room do you have to store a kit?)
2. The purpose of the vessel (offshore cruiser/racer, coastal cruiser, fishing, commercial, charter, etc.)
3. The usual number of people aboard
4. Any significant past or present medical history of the crew
5. Any medications currently taken by any crew member
6. Any previous medical training (i.e., first-aid course, EMT, nurse, etc.) of the crew

In looking for a common denominator to simplify the task of choosing specific items and medications for your vessel's emergency medical kit, I would suggest you place yourself in one of the following categories, based upon the time it *may* take to get to professional medical care:

1. Daysailing/coastal cruising (immediate access to professional medical attention)
2. Coastal cruising (within 1–2 days of professional medical attention)

162

3. Offshore cruising (access to professional medical attention is greater than two days)

Notice that time is used in a relative way (it *may* take one day, or it *may* stretch into a 2–3-day journey because of an unforeseen emergency such as an engine failure or radio malfunction that cuts off all access to anyone). The important thing to remember is that the above categories overlap, and that common sense must be used. In addition, remember to take along any personal medication that a crew member may be taking.

The following examples illustrate the above categories. Modify these recommendations to suit your individual needs.

1. Daysailing/coastal cruising (immediate access to professional medical attention)

Antiseptics/cleansing solution
 PhisoHex
Seasickness
 Transderm-Scōp
 Compazine
Sunburn
 sunscreen with PABA
Burns
 Silvadene
Pain
 aspirin or Tylenol
Bandages and splints
 triangular bandage
 gauze 2 × 2's and 4 × 4's
 adhesive tape
 Ace bandage
 Kling dressing
 butterfly bandages
 eyepads
 Band-Aids
 Telfa pads
Poisoning
 syrup of Ipecac

Appendix 1

2. *Coastal cruising (within 1–2 days of professional medical attention)*

COMPLETE CONTENTS OF KIT I, *PLUS:*
Antibiotics
  ointment
  penicillin, erythromycin
Decongestants
  Sudafed
Cough preparation
  Robitussin
Constipation
  Milk of Magnesia
  Fleet enema
Diarrhea
  Lomotil
  Kaopectate
Earache
  Auralgan drops
  cortisporin drops
Eye medicines
  Sulamyd solution
Pain
  Tylenol #3
Skin rashes
  Tinactin cream
  Monistat-Derm cream
  Calamine lotion
  Benadryl capsules
Toothache
  oil of cloves
Tranquilizer/muscle relaxant
  Valium
Antacid
  Maalox
Snakebite kit
Blood-pressure cuff
Stethoscope

Thermometer
Severe dehydration
  salt tabs

3. Offshore cruising (access to professional medical attention is greater than two days)

COMPLETE CONTENTS OF KITS I AND II, *PLUS:* remaining items listed below that are not listed in KITS I and II (In other words, *Everything! You're on your own out there!*)

The enclosed list states the medication, the strength it is supplied in, and the quantity recommended to take along (in parentheses). Refer to chapter 16.2 for recommended dosages.

ANTIBIOTICS: INFECTIONS

Neosporin or Polymyxin cream or ointment; 15-gram tube, (1) or Bacitracin ointment; ½-oz tube (1)

penicillin or ampicillin, or Keflex; 250–500-mg tablets or capsules (100)

Erythromycin, or tetracycline; 250–500-mg tablet or capsule (100)

Septra; tablets (100) or Septra-DS; tablets (50) Azogantrisin; (60)

Griseofulvin; 250–500-mg tablets (100)

Cortisporin cream or ointment; 7½-gram tube (1)

Mycelex G 1% or Gyne-Lotrimin 1% vaginal cream; 45–90-gram tube (1)

DECONGESTANTS

Sudafed; 60-mg tablet (60)

COUGH PREPARATIONS

Robitussin or Triaminic or Phenergan expectorant; 4–8-oz bottle (1)

Appendix 1

ANTISEPTICS: CLEANSING SOLUTIONS

> PhisoHex, or betadine solution; (1 bottle)
> alcohol; (1 bottle)

CONSTIPATION

> Milk of Magnesia; (1 bottle)
> Fleet enema

DIARRHEA

> Lomotil; (30)
> Imodium; (30)
> Kaopectate; (1 bottle)

EARACHE

> Auralgan; 10-cc bottle (1)
> Cortisporin otic suspension; 10-cc bottle (1)
> Mineral oil

EYE MEDICINES

> Sulamyd-10% ophthalmic; 15-cc bottle (1)
> Neosporin ophthalmic; 10-cc bottle (1)

PAIN RELIEVERS

> Demerol; 50-mg vials or ampules of 2 cc = 100 mg (1–2)
> Morphine; 10 mg/cc vial (1 or 2)
> Tylenol #3 (30)
> Aspirin; 5-grain tablets (60)
> Tylenol (acetaminophen); 325-mg tablets (60)
> Nitroglycerin; $1/_{150}$-grain tablet (100)

SEASICKNESS; SEVERE VOMITING

> Transderm-Scōp; packages of 2 (12)
> Dramamine or Bonine; tablets (30)
> Compazine; 5- or 10-mg tablet or capsule, 2-cc ampules

of 5 mg/cc, or rectal suppository of 25 mg (your choice,
quantity variable)
Tigan; 250-mg capsules, 200-mg ampules, 200-mg rectal
suppositories (your choice, quantity variable)

SKIN RASHES

Tinactin cream or solution 1%; 15-gram tube (1 or 2)
Monistat-Derm cream or lotion; 15-gram tube (1 or 2)
Mycolog cream or ointment; 15-gram tube (1 or 2)
Decadron tablets; 4 mg (30)
Calamine lotion; (1 bottle)
Kwell lotion and shampoo; 2–8 oz bottle (3 each)
Benadryl; 25-mg capsules (30) and vial of 50 mg (1)

BURNS AND SUNBURN

Silvadene cream; 400-gram jar (1)
Sunscreen (your choice; should contain PABA)

TOOTHACHE

Oil of cloves; (1 small bottle)

TRANQUILIZERS: MUSCLE RELAXANTS

Valium; tablets of 2, 5, or 10 mg (30), or 10-cc vial (1)

INSTRUMENTS

Hypodermic syringe; 5–10 cc (3 disposable or 1–2 glass;
several of each would be the best choice). Also, 2–3-
cc disposable ones (2 or 3)
21–23-gauge 1-inch needle (6)
25-gauge $5/8$-inch needle (6)
Suture material; 3-0 and 4-0 ethilon with curved needle
(3 packs)
Urinary catheter (Foley), size 16–18 French (1)
Scissors (1)
Needle driver (1)
Thermometer (2)

Appendix 1

Nasogastric tube, size 16–18 French (1)
Suction bulb
Sterile gloves, small through large (2 or 3)
Clamps (1 or 2)
Tissue forceps (1)
Tweezers (1)
Butterfly needle, 21-gauge (1 or 2)
Safety pins (2)
Magnifying glass (1)

BANDAGES AND SPLINTS

Triangular bandage (sling); (1 or 2)
Gauze bandages; 2 × 2's or 4 × 4's (30)
Telfa pads; (30)
Adhesive tape; 2″ (1 or 2 rolls)
Ace bandage; 2″ and 4″ (1 or 2 of each)
Kling dressing; 3″ (6–12)
Steri-strips; ⅛″ × 3″ (30)
Butterfly bandages; as above
Sterile cotton
Tongue depressors
Sterile eye pads
Splints; various sizes of aluminum or plastic (1 or 2)
Band-Aids (1 box)

POISONING OR OVERDOSE

Syrup of Ipecac; 30-cc bottle (1 or 2)
Narcan; 1-cc ampule of 0.4 mg/cc (2)

MISCELLANEOUS

Epinephrine; 2-cc ampule of 1:1000 (1)
Antacids; Maalox or Mylanta (your choice)
IV's: lactated Ringer's solution and 5% dextrose in water
    solution; 1000-cc bottle (1 or 2)
IV tubing set up (one set)
1% Xylocaine Plain; 50 cc bottle (1–2)
Lasix Tablets; 40 mg, (30)

168

Comprehensive Emergency Medical Kits

Methergine; 0.2 mg, tablets or ampules, (6–8)
Epsom Salts (one package)
Snake Bite Kit (1)
Salt tablets; 500 mg each; 1 bottle of 100
Blood pressure cuff
Stethescope

Appendix 2

Adult Dosages of Common Medications

Caution: Do not take any kind of medication along with any sort of alcoholic beverage (beer, wine, whiskey, etc.).

AURALGAN OTIC

    use: an analgesic used in otitis media (middle ear) infections
    dose: instill drops into affected ear canal every 2–3 hours for pain relief

AZOGANTRISIN

    use: antibiotic used in kidney and bladder infections
    dose: 4 tablets immediately, followed by 2 tablets taken 4 times a day for 10 days

BENADRYL

    use: used in a variety of conditions; including hay fever, allergic reactions, allergic skin disorders (poison ivy, oak, etc.); also motion sickness
    dose:
        orally: 25–50 mg 3–4 times daily
        IM: 25–50 mg 3–4 times daily
    caution: will generally cause fatigue

BONINE

    use: seasickness
    dose: 25–50 mg orally every 24 hours

Adult Dosages of Common Medications

COMPAZINE

   use: the control of severe nausea and vomiting
   dose:
      orally: 5–10-mg tablet or capsule 3–4 times daily
      IM: 5–10 mg 3–4 times daily
      rectal suppository: 25 mg twice daily

CORTISPORIN OTIC SUSPENSION

   use: used in external ear infections (otitis externa)
   dose: 4 drops into the affected ear canal 3–4 times daily
   caution: some people are sensitive to the neomycin contained
in this medication, and react with severe swelling, itching, and
pain to its instillation

DECADRON

   use: many conditions, including severe skin disorders, or allergic reactions
   dose: 1–2 tablet(s) of 4 mg taken daily for the first 5–6 days,
then tapered off by the seventh day

DEMEROL

   use: a very potent narcotic used to relieve pain
   dose: IM, 50–100 mg every 4 hours
   caution: OVERDOSE: Symptoms may include respiratory
depression, cool and clammy skin, and complete circulatory collapse. TREATMENT OF OVERDOSE: CPR if necessary; also,
give the specific narcotic antagonist (antidote) NARCAN, in a
dose of 1–2 ampules (0.4 mg/1cc) IV or IM, IMMEDIATELY)

DRAMAMINE

   use: seasickness
   dose: one 50-mg tablet every 4–6 hours

EPHEDRINE & PROMETHAZINE

   use: seasickness
   dose: variable; consult your personal physician

171

Appendix 2

EPINEPHRINE

use: anaphylactic shock, section 2.4
dose: 0.3–0.5 cc. of 1:1000 solution

GRISEOFULVIN

use: antibiotic useful in treating severe ringworm of the scalp, body, or nails; or very severe athlete's foot
dose: 250–500 mg daily for up to 4 weeks

IMODIUM

use: management of diarrhea
dose: 2 capsules immediately, followed by one capsule after each unformed stool
caution: not to exceed 8 capsules daily

KWELL LOTION & SHAMPOO & CREAM

use: to eradicate scabies, head lice, body lice, crabs
dose: directions for application are on the bottle.

LASIX

use: used as a diuretic to help rid the body of excess fluids
dose: 40 mg orally, IM or IV; usually given 1–2 times daily
caution: diuretic use depletes the body of its stores of cellular potassium, which is necessary for, among other things, the proper functioning of the heart conduction system. An oral potassium supplement may be taken, or eat foods which contain potassium, such as bananas.

LOMOTIL

use: management of diarrhea
dose: 2 tablets up to 4 times a day
caution: not to exceed 8 tablets daily

METHERGINE

use: used during childbirth after the delivery of the placenta to cause uterine bleeding to stop, by causing uterine smooth muscle contraction dose:

    orally: one tablet ($^1/_{320}$ grain) 3–4 times a day for the first 1–2 days after delivery, if needed

    IM: 1 cc ($^1/_{320}$ grain) every 4 hours for the first 1–2 days after delivery, if needed

MONISTAT CREAM OR LOTION

    use: fungal infections of the skin

    dose: apply twice a day to the affected area for 2–4 weeks.

MORPHINE

    use: an extremely potent narcotic used to relieve pain

    dose: given IV in 2-mg increments, up to 10 mg; may be given every 4 hours; if given IM, 5 mg may be given every 4 hours.

    caution: OVERDOSE: SEE TREATMENT OF DEMEROL OVERDOSE, GIVE NARCAN IMMEDIATELY

MYCELEX G 1% or GYNE LOTRIMIN 1% VAGINAL CREAM

    use: antibiotic cream used to treat vaginal yeast infections

    dose: once daily for 7–10 days

MYCOLOG CREAM OR OINTMENT

    use: superficial bacterial, fungal, or yeast infections

    dose: apply to the affected area 2–3 times daily

NARCAN

    use: a specific narcotic antagonist, used when symptoms of narcotic overdose are present

    dose: 1–2 ampules (0.4 mg/1 cc) IM or IV immediately

NEOSPORIN, POLYMYXIN, BACITRACIN CREAM OR OINTMENT

    use: general topical antibacterial

    dose: apply lightly 4 times a day over the affected area

NITROGLYCERIN

    use: the relief of chest pain of cardiac origin, such as angina or acute myocardial infarction (heart attack)

173

dose: one tablet ($^1/_{150}$ grain) placed under the tongue, where it will dissolve spontaneously; may repeat in 5–10 minutes for 2 more times (total of 3 tablets) to relieve chest pain; if the pain persists, give the patient a narcotic such as Demerol or morphine.

PENICILLIN, AMPICILLIN, TETRACYCLINE, ERYTHROMYCIN, KEFLEX

use: antibiotics useful in a variety of infections
dose: orally, 250–500 mg every 6 hours for 7–10 days IM, 300,000–600,000 units every 6 hours of aqueous Procain Penicillin G.

SEPTRA

use: antibiotic used in kidney and bladder infections
dose: 2 tablets every 12 hours for 10 days
note: Septra is also supplied double strength as Septra-DS; dose is one tablet every 12 hours for 10 days.

SILVADENE CREAM

use: antibiotic cream used in second- and third-degree burns
dose: apply twice a day to affected area until healing has occurred

SUDAFED

use: decongestant, used for sinus drainage, cold symptoms, runny nose
dose: 60 mg (one tablet) 3–4 times daily

SULAMYD 10% OPHTHALMIC, NEOSPORIN OPHTHALMIC SOLUTION

use: antibiotic drops used in superficial eye infections
dose: 1–2 drops in the affected eye 4 times daily

SYRUP OF IPECAC

use: to induce vomiting when poisoning or overdose has occurred dose: 15–30 cc (or milliliters) orally, followed by 6–8 glasses of water

caution: causes vomiting; have basin ready! Also, *do not use* in patients who are unconscious, or who have swallowed strong alkalis, acids, or petroleum products (gasoline, etc.)

TIGAN

use: the control of severe nausea and vomiting
dose:
   orally: 250-mg capsule 3–4 times daily
   IM: 200 mg 3–4 times daily
   rectal suppository: 200 mg. 2–4 times daily

TINACTIN 1% CREAM OR SOLUTION

use: fungal infections of the skin
dose: apply twice a day to the affected area for 2–3 weeks

TRANSDERM-SCOP

use: prevention of motion sickness (seasickness)
dose: One unit should be applied to the skin directly behind the ear several hours BEFORE the effect is desired. The effect lasts 72 hours (3 days).

caution: Not to be used by (1) pregnant or nursing mothers, (2) people with glaucoma, (3) people with liver or kidney disease, (4) people with stomach or intestinal problems, (5) people who have trouble urinating, or who have bladder obstructions, and (6) people who have skin allergy or reaction to Scopalamine.

TYLENOL WITH CODEINE

use: for relief of pain
dose: Tylenol #3 has ½ grain of codeine phosphate; Tylenol #4 has one grain of codeine phosphate; 1–2 tablets or capsules taken every 4 hours
caution: OVERDOSE: GIVE NARCAN: SEE ABOVE

Appendix 2

VALIUM

    use: for management of anxiety, severe skeletal muscle spasms, and as an anticonvulsant

    dose:

        orally: 2-, 5-, or 10-mg tablets taken 3–4 times daily

        IM: 5–10 mg 3–4 times daily

Appendix 3

Illness Overseas—Whom to Contact

Illness or injury overseas is an especially difficult situation. A worldwide directory of clinics, hospitals, and English-speaking physicians is available from the following sources; a directory should be obtained prior to departure.

INTERNATIONAL ASSOCIATION FOR MEDICAL
ASSISTANCE TO TRAVELERS

736 Center Street
Lewistown, New York 14092
Telephone: (716) 754-4883

INTERMEDIC

777 Third Avenue
New York, New York 10017
Telephone: (212) 486-8974

UNITED STATES EMBASSIES OR CONSULATES

Staff members may be helpful in directing the person seeking medical aid to local addresses of English-speaking physicians, and in notifying family members in the United States.

If it is necessary to return to the United States for treatment, emergency assistance for air ambulance services is available from these sources:

INTERNATIONAL S.O.S. ASSISTANCE

#1 Neshaminy Interplex, Suite 310
Trevose, Pennsylvania 19047
Telephone: (215) 244-1500

Appendix 3

ASSIST-CARD

745 Fifth Avenue
New York, New York 10022
Telephone: (800) 221-4564 (toll-free)

NEAR, INC.

1900 N. MacArthur Blvd.
Oklahoma City, Oklahoma 73127
Telephone: (800) 654-6060 (toll-free)

COMMERCIAL AIRLINES

Air-ambulance transportation arrangements can be made in most
emergency situations, but may not be available on regular flights,
and expenses may be quite high.

FOR SCUBA OR COMMERCIAL DIVING INJURIES:

Call the DIVERS ALERT NETWORK
Telephone: U.S. (191) 684-2948 or (919) 684-5514 or (919) 684-8111

References

American Red Cross. *Advanced First Aid and Emergency Care*. Garden City: Doubleday & Co., Inc., 1979.

Brunner, Lillan Sholtis, and Suddarth, Doris Smith. *The Lippincott Manual of Nursing Practice*. Philadelphia: J. B. Lippincott Company, 1974.

Center for Disease Control. *Health Information for International Travel*. Atlanta: Public Health Service.

Eastman, Peter F., M.D. *Advanced First Aid Afloat*. Cambridge, MD: Cornell Maritime Press, Inc., 1974.

Haworth, Dr. Robert. *First Aid for Yachtsmen*. London: Adlard Coles Limited, 1975.

Johnson & Johnson. *Professional Uses of Adhesive Tape*. New Brunswick: Johnson & Johnson, 1972.

The Mountaineers. *Medicine for Mountaineering*. Edited by James A. Wilkerson, M.D. Seattle: The Mountaineers, 1975.

Neumann, Hans H., M.D. *Foreign Travel Immunization Guide*. Oradell, NJ: Medical Economics Company Book Division, 1983.

U.S. Department of Health, Education, and Welfare. *The Ship's Medicine Chest and Medical Aid at Sea*. HSA-78-2024 (1978). Washington, D.C.: U.S. Government Printing Office.

Index

Index

Index

Index